AF839928

Pioneer Work in Opening the Medical Profession to Women

Classics in Women's Studies Series

Jane Addams, Emily G. Balch, and Alice Hamilton, *Women at The Hague*

Susan B. Anthony, *The Trial of Susan B. Anthony*

Elizabeth Blackwell, *Pioneer Work in Opening the Medical Profession to Women*

Mary Roberts Coolidge, *Why Women Are So*

Matilda Joslyn Gage, *Woman, Church and State*

Charlotte Perkins Gilman, *The Man-Made World*

Harriet Martineau, *An Independent Woman's Lake District Writings*

Margaret Sanger, *The Pivot of Civilization*

Elizabeth Cady Stanton, *Eighty Years and More*

Mary E. Walker, MD, *Hit: Essays on Women's Rights*

Frances Wright, *Reason, Religion, and Morals*

Pioneer Work in Opening the Medical Profession to Women

Elizabeth Blackwell

WITH AN INTRODUCTION BY

Amy Sue Bix

CLASSICS IN WOMEN'S STUDIES

Humanities Press

ROWMAN & LITTLEFIELD

Lanham • Boulder • New York • London

Published by Rowman & Littlefield
An imprint of The Rowman & Littlefield Publishing Group, Inc.
4501 Forbes Boulevard, Suite 200, Lanham, Maryland 20706
www.rowman.com

86-90 Paul Street, London EC2A 4NE, United Kingdom

Introduction copyright © 2005 by Amy Sue Bix

All rights reserved. No part of this book may be reproduced in any form or by any electronic or mechanical means, including information storage and retrieval systems, without written permission from the publisher, except by a reviewer who may quote passages in a review.

British Library Cataloguing in Publication Information Available

Library of Congress Cataloging-in-Publication Data

The Humanities Press edition of this book was previously catalogued by the Library of Congress as follows:

Blackwell, Elizabeth, 1821-1910.
Pioneer work in opening the medical profession to women : autobiographical sketches / Elizabeth Blackwell ; introduction by Amy Sue Bix.
p. cm. — (Classics in women's studies)
Originally published: London and New York : Longmans, Green and Co., 1895.
Includes bibliographical references.
ISBN 1-59102-255-X (pbk.)
1. Blackwell, Elizabeth, 1821-1910. 2. Women physicians—United States—Biography. [DNLM: 1. Blackwell, Elizabeth, 1821-1910. 2. Physicians, Women—Personal Narratives. WZ 100 B6323p 1895a] I. Title. II. Series.

R692.B576 2004
610'.92—dc22

2004020073

ISBN 9781538179628 (cloth) | ISBN 9781538178355 (pbk.) |
ISBN 9781538178362 (epub)

Physician ELIZABETH BLACKWELL was born on February 3, 1821, at Counterslip, Bristol, England. Her father, Samuel Blackwell, a prosperous sugar refiner, had private tutors educate his children. The Blackwells immigrated to the United States in the summer of 1832, settling in New York City where the family became active in the abolition movement. A few years later, in 1838, shortly after moving the family to Cincinnati, Ohio, Samuel Blackwell died. Elizabeth and two of her sisters helped support the family for several years by operating a boarding school for young women. From 1842 through 1846 she taught school in Kentucky and North and South Carolina.

In 1844, although there was a professional and general prejudice against women doctors, Blackwell began studying medicine privately with sympathetic physicians, and in 1847 she sought formal admission to a medical school. All the leading schools rejected her application, but her persistence paid off and she was finally admitted to the Geneva Medical School—the forerunner of Hobart & William Smith Colleges—in Geneva, New York. In January 1849, ranked first in her class, Blackwell became the first woman in the United States to graduate from medical school.

In April 1849 Blackwell traveled to Europe for advanced studies and practical training. Paris physicians would not permit her to study as a doctor and she was forced to enter the midwives' course at La Maternité, a large maternity hospital. In October 1850 she went to England where she was allowed to continue her studies as a doctor and work at St. Bartholomew's

Hospital. In the summer of 1851 she returned to New York City, where she faced extreme prejudice against women physicians. Her private practice was slow to develop, and she was barred from hospital wards. In the meantime she wrote a series of lectures, published in 1852 as *The Laws of Life, with Special Reference to the Physical Education of Girls.*

In 1853 Blackwell opened a small dispensary in a slum district of New York City, and was eventually joined by her younger sister, Dr. Emily Blackwell, and by Dr. Marie Zakrzewska. The dispensary was enlarged and incorporated as the New York Infirmary for Women and Children in May 1857. During a yearlong lecture tour of Great Britain, in January 1859 Blackwell became the first woman to have her name placed on the British medical register. At the outbreak of the American Civil War, she helped organize the US Sanitary Commission and the Woman's Central Association of Relief, working through the association to train nurses for war service.

In November 1868 Blackwell opened the Woman's Medical College at the infirmary, which would train women as physicians for the next thirty-one years. In 1869 she returned to England where she set up private practice and helped organize the National Health Society in 1871. In 1875 she was appointed professor of gynecology at the London School of Medicine for Women, a position she held until an injury in 1907 forced her to retire. In addition to her lectures, Blackwell authored *The Religion of Health* (1871); *Counsel to Parents on the Moral Education of Their Children* (1878); *The Human Element in Sex* (1884); her autobiography, *Pioneer Work in Opening the Medical Profession to Women* (1895); and *Essays in Medical Sociology* (1902).

Blackwell died on May 31, 1910, at her home in Hastings,

Sussex, England. Since 1949 the American Medical Women's Association has awarded the Elizabeth Blackwell Medal annually to the woman who has made important contributions in advancing the role of women in medicine.

INTRODUCTION

by Amy Sue Bix

The history of women as healers dates back many centuries, long before the life of Elizabeth Blackwell. We have evidence of women as healers and midwives in ancient Greece; for example, some women have funeral inscriptions describing them with the terms "midwife" and "physician." Women's practice of medicine was not universally welcomed; in Athens during the fourth century BCE, female healers were apparently accused of performing illegal abortions and banned from the profession. Stories suggest that one of the era's most famous medical women, Agnodice, had to cut her hair and dress in men's clothing to attend physicians' classes, since her practice of medicine was illegal. Allegedly, when her secret was revealed, Agnodice had won such support among a high-status female clientele that those women blocked their husbands and friends from punishing her. According to some accounts, Agnodice was permitted to continue her work, and the laws were amended to allow women to study and practice medicine as long as they confined their treatments to a female clientele.

In medieval Europe, we have some evidence of women associated around the eleventh century with Salerno, one of the earliest Western centers for medical training. While hostility to women practicing medicine led some countries to ban female healers, Italy proved more open, at least temporarily, especially if women were intending to concentrate on treating female patients. The most famous female figure associated with healing during this era was Trotula, whose name was connected to the production of a highly regarded treatise on gynecology. Trotula may have been both the wife and mother of male physicians, but we know little reliable detail about her.[1]

Medieval women retained a less formal route to enter and perform healing work, providing care for their immediate family and community. These neighborhood healers often built up skill through years of experience and gained a reputation especially for their understanding of herbal cures. The most famous woman associated with herbal medicine during this era is the abbess Hildegard von Bingen, who wrote books setting out lists of folk medicines and described the medical value of hundreds of plants.

Women also served as midwives throughout this period. In some countries, particularly Germany, midwives established their own self-governing profession, training through apprenticeship and agreeing to obey specific rules regulating their work. By 1560 a formal midwifery program had been established in Paris. Unfortunately, there were also episodes of suspicion attached to female healers, especially during Europe's "witchcraft craze" of the 1400s, 1500s, and 1600s. In an era when both the church and popular superstition perceived women as credulous and weak in character—easy prey for the temptations of the devil—a midwife might be blamed for a baby's death, collecting its soul for Satan.

This tradition of women as community healers and midwives extended into colonial America. Especially in rural areas or on the frontier, where access to any other medical care was difficult, the job of tending the sick was handled within the family and primarily considered woman's responsibility. In fact, colonial America did not really have an established, separate medical profession as we recognize it today; it was considered normal for laypeople to dispense medical services, relying on common sense, folk remedies, and herbal cures. Those who did establish a physician's practice could do so without being required to earn a medical degree. Many eighteenth-century physicians trained by apprenticeship, learning by serving as assistant to an established doctor and reading his medical books. After about three years, the apprentice might be judged to have reached proficiency, but there were no outside examinations, no national standards. America's first medical school did not appear until 1765, and at the time of the Revolution, only about one out of ten physicians practicing in the United States held an MD degree.

The decades after the Revolution brought many changes in American life, including for women. Back in the colonial era, white women occupied a socially and intellectually circumscribed role, legally considered dependents on the men of their families. Tradition and necessity tied most to an unending daily routine of demanding domestic chores, leaving them little time and few recognized avenues for involvement in anything other than home and church. Tradition and commonly held assumptions reserved the public sphere of government and politics for men. Even in relatively literate New England, girls had less access to education than boys; large numbers of women were never even taught to write.[2]

While the Revolution did not instantly alter American

women's subordinate legal status or give them political recognition as citizens with equal rights, subsequent years did see a new rhetorical importance attached to women's traditional roles. Authors, ministers, and other observers promoted a set of ideas that historians have called "Republican Motherhood," which emphasized women's responsibility as guardians of children and society, nurturing patriotic and moral virtues. The basic principle suggested that the best way for women to contribute to the newly independent nation was not to vote or earn money, but to concentrate on shaping their sons into good citizens and their daughters into proper future mothers. The idea implied that the home served a national public function, that while staying within domestic life, women could exert important influence over children, husbands, and by extension the nation, maintaining society's purity and strength.[3]

Republican Motherhood offered some justification for expanding women's education; in order to instill religious principles, moral values, and some basic knowledge of fields like mathematics and geography in children, women would need solid grounding in those areas themselves. Reformers such as Judith Sargent Murray argued for giving girls new access to learning, to expand their minds, develop their self-respect, and provide the tools to give them self-sufficiency if they were widowed or otherwise left without a man's support.

During the early 1800s, American education for both boys and girls expanded. Public schools were created in major cities, while private schools, separated by gender, were established in Philadelphia, Boston, and smaller towns. There was no standardized curriculum, but innovators such as Emma Willard created academies that reflected a broadened view of what young women should learn. Reaching beyond practical subjects such as needlework and beyond "ornamental" instruction in music, drawing, and other feminine graces, these academies often included classes in history, literature, and other substantive fields. The intent was not to turn girls into scholarly grinds, distracting them from women's traditional path of family and domesticity; precisely the opposite. Advocates argued that properly oriented education would make young women better wives and mothers, more fit to raise children and manage a household well.

Upon finishing school, many young women did indeed get married; middle-class women had few other commonly accepted avenues in life. However, one area of opportunity attracted an increasing number; after acquiring some education, women could become teachers. As westward settlement expanded and more schools opened, demand for teachers rose, and towns could hire female teachers at a fraction of a man's cost. Teaching offered women a valuable chance to become wage earners, supporting themselves or contributing to family financial resources. The rationale for having female teachers extended the rhetoric of Republican Motherhood, suggesting that women possessed an innate gentleness and patience that made them a natural influence on children.[4] By the 1850s, one out of approximately every five white women in Massachusetts had taught school at some point in her lifetime, and the ranks of nineteenth-century female teachers includes such well-known names as Susan B. Anthony, Carrie Chapman Catt, and Elizabeth Blackwell.[5]

Advocates such as Catharine Beecher promoted the transformation of teaching into a woman's profession. Beecher hoped that just as men entered medicine or law, women would find "true and noble" work in teaching, a path that could "elevate and dignify" women without encroaching on male territory. Far from undermining natural femininity, she argued, teaching would enhance it, developing women's characters. Beecher hoped that by drawing on their strengths of purity and piety, female teachers would become "a new source of moral power" in their towns, inculcating thrift, order, and virtue in students, and by extension rescuing the nation from ignorance and vice. During the 1840s, Beecher raised money to recruit new female teachers; setting up her own teacher-training institute, she dispatched over four hundred women to new schoolhouses, particularly on the frontier.[6]

While Beecher portrayed teaching as a natural feminine occupation, female teachers also broke new ground by leaving home, earning money, and holding highly visible public positions in their communities. These women, especially on the frontier, found adventure, challenges, and a certain independence simply in traveling to new areas, often in still-rough territory. As single women, however, teachers were also constrained by gender expectations and paternalistic chaperoning; their behavior was closely observed, and the life of boarding with a strange family could prove lonely and difficult.

Especially for upper-middle-class women, the early nineteenth century brought a phenomenon that historians have called the "cult of domesticity" or the "cult of true womanhood." Religious leaders, books, and other sources promoted the idea that man's place was naturally in public life, woman's in private. In an era when the world of business and politics seemed increasingly stressful, writers emphasized that women should make the home a sacred refuge, an emotional center to reinforce the morality under threat by outside corruption. The idea that women must safeguard the family (and by extension, the community and nation) encouraged the already common tendency to define women's and men's natures as opposites. If men were competitive and individualistic, women should be cooperative and self-sacrificing, inhabiting a more noble sphere. Advice manuals encouraged girls to cultivate soft feminine virtues such as modesty, docility, delicacy, tenderness, cheerfulness, and sympathy. This rhetoric of "separate spheres" lent domesticity new emotional weight (though not financial; women's housework remained unpaid), reinforcing the expectations of women to meet ideals of purity and piety.

Ironically, beliefs connecting women to a higher moral plane ended up creating an avenue for some to move outside narrow domestic life. The early 1800s brought a religious reawakening in the United States, which in turn promoted campaigns against alcohol, prostitution, and slavery. The idea of wives, mothers, and teachers as moral guardians gave them a justification to participate in these social reform movements. Some estimates suggest that women comprised more than half the membership of abolition societies during the 1830s, for example.

Involvement with such causes gave women experience speaking in public and performing other new activities, built connections between sympathetic and energetic men and women, and, among some women, raised consciousness of injustice in American democracy. Offended by rules barring them, as female delegates, from publicly participating in a major antislavery conference, abolition supporters Lucretia Mott and Elizabeth Cady Stanton noticed the irony of denying women representation at a meeting talking about freedom and human rights. In 1848 in Seneca Falls, New York, Mott and Stanton organized the first meeting specifically convened to address women's rights as a social and political issue. The convention issued a "Declaration of Sentiments," modeled after the Declaration of Independence, listing women's grievances of their secondary legal, social, and educational status. The more than two hundred women (plus several dozen men) attending adopted resolutions calling for increasing women's opportunities in life. The most controversial proposal was female suffrage; the concept of women voting remained far too radical, sounding strange and outrageous even to most women. The Seneca Falls convention met ridicule and denunciation from churches and the press, but inspired other women to organize meetings to continue discussing women's place in American life.

During these decades, women who wanted the right to vote, women who gave antislavery speeches in public, and women who otherwise seemed to go too far in challenging the ideal of separate spheres had to be prepared for criticism, scorn, and ridicule. Attacks extended to the continuing advance of women's education. In 1842 Oberlin became the first college to present degrees to women, and by the 1870s state colleges such as Iowa, Wisconsin, and Michigan were admitting female students. This period also brought the creation of women's colleges, starting with the 1837 opening of Mount Holyoke in South Hadley, Massachusetts. Self-educated herself, founder Mary Lyon wanted to create a school to offer other young women intellectual opportunity, personal growth, and a chance to contribute to society. Lyon particularly hoped to turn out what she called "self-denying female teachers,"[7] and indeed, more than 80 percent of pre-1850 graduates taught school for at least some time.

The other "Seven Sisters" (Vassar, Wellesley, Smith, Bryn Mawr, Radcliffe, and Barnard) were established between 1860 and 1890, and by 1891 over ten thousand women were enrolled in higher education, in both coeducational and all-women settings.

Yet even as women's opportunities for higher education grew, the concept of women pursuing advanced study remained controversial in many quarters. Colleges had traditionally aimed to prepare men for the legal or theological professions or for work as enlightened farmers or mechanics; there seemed scarce rationale for encouraging women to master Latin or science. Indeed, the fear was that women entering college like men might become too much like men, losing their uniquely feminine virtues. Leaders of women's colleges were placed on the defensive, asserting repeatedly that their institutions would cultivate, not destroy, women's nature. Vassar insisted that its college life was grounded in a wholesome, protective community, ensuring that education would not "impair womanliness in our students & encourage the formation of those mannish tastes and manners which are so disgusting to every right mind." In establishing her college, Sophie Smith declared, "It is not my design to render my sex any the less feminine, but to develop as fully as may be the powers of womanhood and furnish women with means of usefulness, happiness and honor now withheld from them."[8]

Critics warned that higher education risked "desexing" women, not only in character, but in body. Science of the late eighteenth and early nineteenth centuries emphasized sexual differences in anatomy and physiology, pronouncing that nature had shaped women's skeletons, minds, and character specifically for the purpose of reproduction. Such scientific evidence seemed to support older church teachings that divine purpose imbued men with physical and intellectual strength, women with capacity for motherhood.[9] Anatomists emphasized the childbearing function of the female pelvis, while anthropologists and craniologists pointed to women's smaller brains. Darwinism linked maleness to evolution of cleverness and daring, while suggesting that females were more primitive, merely passing along the species through reproduction.[10]

Such assumptions also shaped medical thought and treatment. For centuries, observers had often assumed that the female reproductive system must be the primary factor governing women's health. Following the philosophy of Aristotle, the ancient Greek physician Galen idealized men as the true and normal type of human, with women as comparatively incomplete and flawed, physically and intellectually. Some medical thought in ancient Greece indicated that the womb ("hystera") could become displaced and literally wander around a woman's body, causing all sorts of illnesses.[11] Hippocratic writings warned that young girls at the onset of puberty were especially vulnerable, reporting cases of suicidal insanity in virgins. Assumptions that women were by nature more emotional and less rational than men were carried into later centuries, reinforced by superstition and the misogyny of church authorities. Nineteenth-century diagnoses of "hysteria" often reflected continuing assumptions that women were emotionally, mentally, and physically weaker than men.

Nineteenth-century thought, science, and medicine frequently defined women's biology in terms of their reproductive capacity, a tendency echoing "separate spheres" ideology's emphasis on motherhood. One doctor in 1870 declared that it was "as if the Almighty, in creating the female sex, had taken the uterus and built up a woman around it."[12]

Medical wisdom regarded the proper development of the reproductive system in young women as a key concern. The onset of menstruation was seen as a time placing great strain on the female body. Popular health manuals urged women to recognize their menstrual-cycle weaknesses, noting, "We cannot too emphatically urge the importance of regarding these monthly returns as periods of ill health, when ordinary occupations are to be suspended or modified. Long walks, dancing, shopping, riding and parties should be avoided." Women's biology was interpreted as poised on the edge of sickness; in 1900, one of America's most prominent gynecologists declared, "Many a young life is battered and forever crippled on the breakers of puberty; if it crosses these unharmed and is not dashed to pieces on the rock of childbirth, it may still ground on the ever-recurring shadows of menstruation, and lastly upon the final bar of the menopause ere protection is found in the unruffled waters of the harbor beyond reach of sexual storms."[13] Of course, nineteenth-century women did face appallingly high risks of dying from complications of childbirth. Among other very real causes of health problems, corsets and heavy garments exerted substantial pressure on internal organs and constrained movement. Women told that they should retire from the outside world might begin expecting to collapse each menstrual period. But more than that, assumptions that upper-class women by nature were especially delicate contributed to the romanticization of graceful illness and a fashionable image of the fragile woman.[14]

Analogies commonly compared a body to an economic system, with a limited amount of resources; women who devoted too much attention to mental exercise thus risked draining vital energy away from their reproductive organs.[15]

Harvard Professor of Material Medica Edward Clarke warned that women should not be allowed to endanger their future role as wives and mothers by studying as hard as men did. Clarke wrote, "Girls lose health, strength, blood, and nerve, by a regimen that ignores the periodical tides and reproductive apparatus of their organization. . . . [I]dentical education of the two sexes is a crime before God and humanity, that physiology protests against and experience weeps over."[16] Clarke and other critics cited cases of women whose college education supposedly caused headaches, menstrual irregularities, and more serious problems including insanity and infertility.

Such warnings made a real impact, causing some people to have serious doubts about women's education. Activists fought back, collecting evidence that college-educated women enjoyed excellent health and promoting what one historian has called "able-bodied womanhood," the idea that women could be strong and even enjoy activities such as bicycling and team sports.[17]

The idea that women were by nature weaker and more emotional than men, suited by nature for motherhood and morality, reinforced "separate sphere" arguments that women had no place in traditionally male work. During the nineteenth century, the practice of medicine had become contested territory, a complex social and economic conflict over who had the power to claim knowledge and exert expert authority. Different Americans received medical care from different sources; wealthy urban patients could patronize elite doctors who had been able to afford formal medical training, perhaps even pursuing postgraduate studies with advanced practitioners in Europe. Poorer families might treat themselves with the help of home medical-advice manuals, consult the neighborhood healer or midwife, or go to self-taught doctors or those who learned through apprenticeship, along with "bone setters," "bleeders," herbalists, and purveyors of commercial remedies.

During this period, there were wide disagreements over what constituted "proper" forms of treatment for disease. Allopathic or "regular" medical care called for practitioners to treat disease aggressively, using "heroic measures" such as bloodletting, purging, blistering, or heavy doses of poisonous substances such as mercury. Doctors defined the violent nature of these procedures as proof of their efficacy, dramatically reflecting the struggle to conquer disease and force it out of the body. However, the physical toll exerted aroused fear and mistrust among some observers, especially when physicians failed to save patients. Critics in the 1830s and 1840s warned that many people barely escaped with their lives after being "butchered by Pill givers" and poisoned with mercury-based calomel. Such concerns encouraged sectarianism, the promotion of alternative philosophies of illness and healing.[18]

Some varieties of alternative medicine attracted women's interest precisely because they promised more gentle treatment and stressed preventative measures.[19] Elizabeth Cady Stanton, Susan B. Anthony, Louisa May Alcott, Harriet Beecher Stowe, Catharine Beecher, and Julia Ward Howe, among other notables, favored various irregular treatments. Some forms of alternative medicine also supported political and social causes that appealed to many women, including "dress reform."[20] Hydropathy practitioners often denounced tight corseting, for example.[21] Hydropathic specialists, who fought disease with cold baths and other water treatments, attracted a prominent midcentury clientele, including Anthony and Beecher. Modesty dictated that female patients undergoing immersion should be attended by female staff, and thus, for reasons of propriety, hydropathy welcomed women practitioners. Some historians have suggested that women comprised from one-fifth to one-third of hydropathic practitioners, although men claimed the highest ranks as spas' chief physicians.[22]

In general, sectarian approaches opened certain opportunities for women to practice medicine. During the second half of the 1800s, many schools of alternative medicine embraced coeducation as both a practical measure and philosophical statement. Hundreds of women attended New York's homeopathic Women's Medical College, the eclectic Penn Medical University, and the American Hydropathic Institute. Some entered sectarian schools out of necessity when their access to allopathic education was blocked; others were drawn by ideological commitment to nature cures.[23] The American Institute of Homeopathy (AIH) voted to accept female members in 1869, forty-six years before the American Medical Association officially changed its bylaws to permit women's admission. Female homeopaths served as delegates to AIH annual meetings and were chosen to hold local and national offices. More than that, women constituted a clear majority of homeopathic patients, and advocates looked to the continuation and expansion of this female constituency to help their beleaguered cause remain alive into the twentieth century.[24]

Women might enjoy a certain access to study and practice alternative medicine, but their opportunities were still limited by gender expectations and by practical constraints such as money for tuition. More than that, this fact only underlined the barriers blocking women's participation in allopathic medicine. Between about 1810 and 1880, a number of new medical schools had been established in both cities and rural areas. Such institutions generally did not offer students laboratories, libraries, or hospital experience. Schools run for profit competed to attract students, encouraging a looseness of standards; admission to medical school did not require a college diploma or any other substantial prerequisites. Professors who got paid only if students passed tended to make examinations easy. Still, common assumptions limited training to men.

Opposition to allowing women into mainstream medicine rested partly on the opinion voiced by Edward Clarke, among many others, that the demands of the female reproductive system meant women simply did not have the physical stamina or the proper mental abilities for studying or practicing medicine. Critics pointed to women's supposed emotional instability, hinting at the frightening prospect of female surgeons performing operations while displaying the weakness and mental fluctuations accompanying menstruation. They argued that female doctors would not be able to travel safely or conveniently at night to treat medical emergencies, and that it would be impractical and wrong for women to try to combine medical practice with marriage and children.[25]

Even more important, critics argued that medical training was simply inappropriate for women, touching on vulgar subjects that no decent lady should even want to consider. Clarke said, "God forbid I should ever see men and women aiding each other to display with the scalpel the secrets of the reproductive system or charmingly discuss syphilis together." Idealization of women as gentle and refined (despite the fact that in practice, motherhood involved plenty of messy and difficult situations) led one gynecologist to say in 1892, "Medicine is disgusting to women accustomed to the soft side of life."

Critics warned that medical study would destroy natural feminine delicacy and purity by exposing them to risqué jokes about intimate matters and demanding that they dissect bodies.

In an 1820 argument that more clearheaded male practitioners should replace female midwives in attending births, Harvard medical professor Walter Channing warned against such coarsening: "[I]t is obvious that we cannot instruct women as we do men in the science of medicine; we cannot carry them into the dissecting room and the hospital; many of our more delicate feelings, much of our refined sensibility must be subdued, before we can submit to the sort of discipline required in the study of medicine; in females they must be destroyed."[26] There were negative connotations attached to the image of female physicians, making them seem less than respectable, partly because infamous abortionist Madam Restell was referred to as a "doctor."

Quite simply, women who expressed interest in medicine were perceived as freaks, violating women's natural domestic orientation and seeking to become like men. In the *Boston Medical and Surgical Journal* of 1850, one doctor commented,

> I am unqualifiedly opposed to educating females for the medical profession. . . . [T]hey are not constituted for an employment of this character. . . . [T]here is a vast difference, a wide "gulf" in the instinctive faculties, tastes and propensities of the two sexes, and which declare to each . . . "thus far and no farther shalt thou go." . . . The bare mention of the thought of married females engaging in the medical profession is too palpably absurd to require any exposition. It carries . . . a sense of shame, vulgarity and disgust. . . . To the female sex . . . may

> be attributed the *nervous* or *excitable* temperament. . . . [I]n a profession where the *utmost nerve* and *self-possession* are often required, the male sex is the most favorably constituted. . . . [I]t is in the domestic circle that woman's talents and virtues display themselves with the greatest brilliancy. . . . [S]he must be content to labor in her sphere. . . . [W]hen she aspires to be the *competitor* of man, she must abandon all claim to the love, sympathy and affection which are so freely bestowed upon her. . . . [L]et woman not assume the prerogatives of *man*, by entering the arena and noisy business of life, for which she has not faculties in common with *man*.[27]

For some male doctors, opposition to allowing women to practice may have been at least partly a reaction to fears of professional competition. By the mid-1800s, multiplication of practitioners had left the field overcrowded, with many struggling to remain solvent or forced to supplement medical income with other jobs. There was fear that female patients particularly might choose to patronize female doctors, especially for intimate problems. During the 1870s, the *Boston Medical Journal* published a poem roughly translated as, "And when the ladies get degrees, depend on it there's nothing will please, til they have got our chairs and fees, and there's an end of you and me."[28]

The obstacles facing women are illustrated by the case of Harriot Hunt, born in 1805 to a middle-class family. When her sister became ill, standard treatments of bleeding and blistering seemed to bring little improvement and appalled Hunt. In desperation, the family turned to botanical medicine, where practitioners also seemed less intimidating. Hunt apprenticed herself to those alternative physicians and in 1835 set up her own medical office in Boston. Realizing the advantage that a medical degree gave a practitioner, Hunt applied to Harvard Medical College in 1847, with the hope that her previous experience gave her credibility. After an initial rejection, Harvard officials considered letting Hunt attend lectures, but in the end, that possibility was blocked by student protests that having a woman in medical classes would be awkward, immoral, and impair the dignity of the school. Hunt continued practicing medicine in Boston for over twenty-five years, gradually building her clientele and delivering lectures to instruct women about their bodies and hygiene.[29]

This was the context within which Elizabeth Blackwell struggled and ultimately succeeded in becoming the first woman to receive an MD from an allopathic medical school. As her autobiography relates, she was born near Bristol, England in 1821 into a large, socially conscious family that took learning seriously, for daughters as well as sons. For economic and ideological reasons, the Blackwells moved to the United States when Elizabeth was eleven. First in the New York City area and then in Cincinnati, the family environment was immersed in liberal politics and high culture, with William Lloyd Garrison, Harriet Beecher Stowe, and William Henry Channing as family acquaintances. After her father's death, family financial difficulties led Elizabeth and other daughters to run a boarding school. While Elizabeth subsequently left home for teaching positions in Kentucky, North Carolina, and South Carolina, she was increasingly absorbed by a desire to study medicine. Since Blackwell admitted a dislike for disease, this plan did not represent a natural choice, but rather an intriguing moral challenge and divinely inspired obligation to work for social progress. Blackwell was allegedly also spurred by a female friend dying of cancer, who said she would have been more comfortable seeing a female doctor rather than strange men.

Given the strong revulsion in so many quarters to the very idea of women in medicine, it becomes clearer to see why a number of doctors whom Blackwell consulted were doubtful about her chance of acceptance or suggested that she disguise herself in male garb. It should also not prove surprising that Blackwell's applications to major medical schools in New York, Philadelphia, and elsewhere were rejected. Her admission to New York's Geneva College appears to have been a fluke; the faculty referred the question of accepting Blackwell to the student body, perhaps as a handy excuse to reject her. The students seem to have regarded the situation as a prank, perhaps by a rival college, and so agreed to admit a woman. When Blackwell actually showed up, her reception among fellow students, faculty, and townspeople was uneven, with some offering acceptance and even support, others amazement or hostility, as her autobiography relates. Blackwell received her MD in January 1849 after completing a thesis on ship fever and typhus that focused on the role of sanitation in fighting disease, the need for social reform as part of health care, and the aim of relieving suffering in individual patients. Her degree proved controversial; the American Medical Association, established in 1847, initially censured Geneva Medical College. Though that decision was later reversed, Geneva subsequently refused for a number of years to accept any more female students, rejecting Elizabeth's sister Emily among others.[30]

Like many ambitious and intellectually curious male medical graduates who could manage it, Blackwell was interested in obtaining postgraduate training in Europe, where medical centers with a worldwide reputation for medical excellence drew students from all over. It was easier for young practitioners to gain a large amount of practical clinical experience and postmortem dissection in Paris than in the United States.[31] But after doctors proved skeptical about a woman's chances of gaining access to work in major general hospitals, Blackwell ended up joining the midwives' program at La Maternité, Europe's largest obstetrics hospital. After an accident in practice led to infection that cost Blackwell part of her vision, she completed her training in England, where she became friends with prominent social reformers and many leading medical figures, including Florence Nightingale.

In the summer of 1851 Blackwell returned to New York, where she immediately experienced difficulty establishing her medical practice. She was barred from city hospitals (even from the women's wards), unable to rent good space to live and work, and even allegedly received anonymous hate letters. During this time, Blackwell delivered a set of lectures on women's anatomy and girls' health (published in 1852 as *The Laws of Life, with Special Reference to the Physical Education of Girls*); some women in the audience were apparently won over to support Blackwell's work.

Given her professional isolation from existing medical institutions, Blackwell moved to start her own dispensary on New York's East Side in 1853. Poor immigrants without any other access to good medical care flocked to Blackwell's clinic, soon known as the New York Infirmary for Women and Children. In addition to treating the needy, Blackwell made it her institution's mission to give other female physicians a place to practice. Elizabeth was soon joined by her sister Emily and her friend Marie Zakrzewska (both graduates of Cleveland Medical College of Western Reserve College), making the New York Infirmary the first hospital staffed by female doctors. Emily had received postgraduate training in prestigious Edinburgh. Zakrzewska, born in Berlin in 1829, had excelled at medical school and been appointed chief midwife and professor in Prussia's school for midwives. Upon coming to the United States in 1853, she realized that she would have a better chance of success with an American medical degree. With the encouragement and financial assistance of Blackwell and other women, Zakrzewska returned to school.[32]

In the years since Elizabeth first tried to enter medical school, a few small windows of opportunity had opened for other women. In 1848 the New England Female Medical College (NEFMC) opened, the world's first medical school for women. To minimize controversy, founders planned for their graduates to confine their practice to women and children, which they also considered the natural and best path for female doctors. The school promised to maintain "that nice sense of delicacy which is the ornament of the female character, the soul of virtue and the safeguard of morals." Unfortunately, the NEFMC had few financial resources, its facilities were weak, and the school was unable to be very selective in admissions. Many in Boston's medical community opposed the school, refusing to let its students work in city hospitals. The school graduated some women who set up successful practices (including the first African American woman to earn a medical degree), but collapsed in the early 1870s.[33] However, in the meantime, liberal-minded Philadelphians had opened the Women's Medical College of Pennsylvania in 1850. During the school's first graduation, male medical students allegedly threatened to disrupt proceedings, and the school called policemen for protection.

Ann Preston, who graduated in the first class and subsequently became physiology professor and dean at the college, continued the fight to justify women's study of medicine. After the Philadelphia County Medical Society instructed its members to not associate with female doctors, she wrote an essay calling women's medical training an "inevitable" part of modern progress, giving women the right to exercise their God-given talents. Indeed, she pointed out, countless women had already demonstrated their ability to tend the sick "with a power of sustained endurance that man does not even claim to possess." Preston continued,

> Our position is womanly, that this work is established in the fitness of things. . . . On behalf of a little band of true-hearted young women who are just entering the profession . . . we must protest . . . against the injustice which places difficulties in our way, not because we are ignorant or pretentious or incompetent . . . but because we are women.[34]

Blackwell argued in an 1860 speech that still more women should become doctors, in order to spread knowledge about physiology and sanitation to mothers and teachers, thereby helping them raise healthy children and maintain household and community health. She said,

> The application of scientific knowledge to women's necessities in actual life can only be done by women who possess at once the scientific learning of the physician, and as women a thorough acquaintance with women's requirements. . . . [Male] physicians are too far removed from women's life; they can criticize but not guide it. . . . The fact that more than half

> of ordinary medical practice lies among women and children, would seem to be . . . proof enough that there must be here a great deal that women could do.[35]

In 1864 Blackwell declared that now that other women had joined her in earning degrees and beginning medical work, "the practice of medicine by women is no longer a doubtful, but a settled thing," and yet "there is not in the whole . . . country a single medical school where women can obtain a good medical education." She worried that existing opportunities for training were inadequate, insufficiently rigorous, and hampered by lack of funds. Accordingly, Blackwell planned to start her own school and officially opened the Woman's Medical College of New York Infirmary in 1868. Concerned with educational quality, Blackwell required a total of fifteen to twenty months of study, when many other schools considered ten or twelve months sufficient. Blackwell declared that her college would be the world's first to create a chair of hygiene, and she became the first professor to fill that post.[36]

Meanwhile, Elizabeth had undertaken other significant work. In 1859 she visited England again, where she delivered lectures on the state of American health care and encouraged British women interested in medicine to contact her. She told them,

> Though a woman may now become a legally qualified practitioner of medicine, the task is still a very arduous one. . . . Society has not yet recognized this study as fit woman's work. Gossip and slander may annoy the student, and . . . the absence of social and professional support . . . [make it] a long and difficult struggle. There is a noble and useful life to be

> gained by the conquest of these difficulties, but . . . they require perseverance, courage, and self-reliance.[37]

Soon after her return to New York in 1860, with the onset of the Civil War, Blackwell became caught up in the problem of addressing urgent military medical needs. The army had no established arrangements to provide systematic care and had no facilities. Military medicine conditions were outdated, inadequate, or even nonexistent. Many soldiers living in filthy camps succumbed to contagious disease, while wounded men might be left dying on the battlefield for hours or even days. After a meeting convened in 1861 at the Blackwells' infirmary, Elizabeth and Emily helped lead efforts to provide military medical care. Their organization, the Women's Central Relief Association (WCRA), helped to recruit skilled women as nurses and give them proper training. This voluntary effort drew on Florence Nightingale's model, especially her emphasis on hospital cleanliness and patient hygiene. The WCRA's efforts helped lead to the establishment of the United States Sanitary Commission, predecessor to the American Red Cross.[38]

The New York Infirmary kept growing; in 1865 it treated over thirty thousand patients.[39] But in 1869, Elizabeth returned to England for good, where her medical practice drew patients from her wide circle of acquaintances. She also lectured, wrote, and worked to expand access to medical education and practice for women in England.[40] Together with Elizabeth Garrett Anderson and Sophia Jex Blake, Blackwell helped establish the London School of Medicine for Women in 1874 and held the chair of gynecology there until her own illness cut that short. She argued that overall health conditions would be improved by having more female doctors since women were best positioned to understand family medical issues and, by extension, society health needs. While many male doctors could exhibit sympathy, she said, women were by nature more empathetic and predisposed to care for others.[41] In an 1890 address to the London School of Medicine for Women, Blackwell said,

> Women are called upon very specially to judge all practical action as right or wrong. . . . It is through the moral, guiding the intellectual, that the beneficial influence of women in any new sphere of activity will be felt. . . . [W]omen from their constitutional adaptation to creation and guardianship, are thus fitted for a special and noble part in the advancement of the healing art.[42]

Toward Blackwell's later life, the direction of medicine was undergoing significant change. Her education at midcentury had emphasized treating sickness in a holistic manner, where health was regarded as a continually adjusted state of balance within body, whose parts all interacted, and between body and environment. Disease was understood as a disturbance of equilibrium, for which individualized treatment should reflect a physician's understanding of the patient's specific condition and family background, plus environmental factors such as season and climate.[43] But especially after the 1870s, major new discoveries in bacteriology and immunology gave new power to laboratory-based medical science. The germ theory of disease promised to place ideas about illness on a new foundation of objectivity by identifying specific microorganisms as causes of cholera, typhoid fever, tuberculosis, and other serious diseases. While Blackwell certainly respected science, she felt uncomfortable with this new materialist, mechanistic approach to disease. She and other critics feared that an obsession with isolating microbes could distract from the need for doctors to cultivate a sympathetic relationship with the patient, aimed at easing their suffering. Blackwell also worried that laboratory science risked cutting off awareness of the many social factors contributing to disease, especially sanitary problems. Blackwell also felt disturbed by experimentation on animals and became active in antivivisection campaigns.[44] She considered it unethical to cause living creatures pain even in pursuit of knowledge and worried that such inhumane practices would blunt doctors' capacity for sympathy.[45]

For Blackwell, medicine represented part of a commitment to social reform and moral uplift. She had grown up in a politically progressive family, active in the abolition movement. One of her brothers married early feminist and abolitionist Lucy Stone while another married Antoinette Brown, America's first formally ordained female minister.[46] Elizabeth herself actively participated in her era's moral reform movement, joining the campaign to fight prostitution and citing her medical experience in pointing to its harmful effects on health and morality.

Blackwell also continued writing, producing an 1879 book on sex education so scandalous that publishers refused it until a group of clergymen approved the topic and suggested a more discreet title.[47] Blackwell also maintained her commitment to the sanitary movement and to promoting health awareness among the general public; she helped create Britain's National Health Society in 1871. Elizabeth Blackwell died in England in 1910 at age eighty-nine.

During her lifetime, conditions facing women who wished

to enter medicine in the United States had improved in significant ways. According to some historians, it is no coincidence that women gained new access to medical training during the same time as the rise of the women's rights movement. Feminism offered moral and psychological support for women doctors, as well as tangible backing in the form of fund-raising. Indeed, feminist leaders helped induce the Johns Hopkins Medical School to admit women, in exchange for a donation of several hundred thousand dollars. By the 1890s Cornell, Michigan, Iowa, and several other medical schools had become coeducational. By 1900 there were an estimated seven thousand women practicing medicine, with roughly one-third to one-half of them holding some type of degree. Female doctors were publishing books and articles, setting up their own medical journals and professional societies.[48] In 1902 anatomist Florence Sabin became the first female faculty member at Johns Hopkins Medical School, and Alice Hamilton, who pioneered in developing the field of industrial medicine, was named to Harvard's public health faculty in 1918. During WWI, American female doctors ran an overseas hospital on behalf of the French government since the US Army accepted female nurses but refused women doctors' efforts to volunteer for service. To varying extents, women still faced hostility and teasing in the course of daily medical lectures and hospital routine, plus discrimination in finding internships and employment, gaining access to facilities, and receiving fair treatment.[49] Moreover, even as schools such as Michigan began admitting women, some of the old female medical colleges collapsed under financial strain or merged with other institutions. With the marginalization of alternative medicine, many homeopathic medical schools that had accepted women were shut. Between 1902 and 1926, the number of female medical students actually fell. The later twentieth century brought significant change, however. Especially in the 1970s, under the influence of the feminist movement and affirmative action, numbers of female medical students in the United States began rising from post–World War II lows. Between 1959–60 and 1976, the number of women entering medical school grew more than 700 percent. By 1975–76, women comprised almost 21 percent of all enrolled medical students. The years 2002–2004 represented the first time ever that the number of women applying to medical school exceeded the number of men, a fact that surely would have intrigued Elizabeth Blackwell.[50]

Amy Sue Bix
Associate Professor
Program in the History of Technology and Science
Iowa State University

NOTES

The author wishes to thank Dr. Alan Marcus and Cai Guise-Richardson for their assistance in preparing this piece.

1. Margaret Alic, *Hypatia's Heritage: A History of Women in Science from Antiquity through the Nineteenth Century* (Boston: Beacon Press, 1986).

2. Nancy Woloch, *Women and the American Experience* (Boston: McGraw Hill, 2000).

3. Linda K. Kerber, "The Republican Mother: Women and the Enlightenment, an American Perspective," *American Quarterly* 28 (Summer 1976): 187–205; and Linda K. Kerber, *Toward an Intellectual History of Women* (Chapel Hill: University of North Carolina Press, 1997).

4. Barbara Miller Solomon, *In the Company of Educated Women: A History of Women and Higher Education in America* (New Haven, CT: Yale University Press, 1985).

5. Maris A. Vinovskis and Richard M. Bernard, "The Female Schoolteacher in Antebellum Massachusetts," *Journal of Social History* 10 (March 1977): 332–45.

6. Kathryn Kish Sklar, *Catharine Beecher: A Study in American Domesticity* (New Haven, CT: Yale University Press, 1973).

7. Woloch, *Women and the American Experience,* p. 132.

8. *Smith College Bulletin: Catalogue no. 1960–61* (Northhampton, MA: Smith College, 1960).

9. Nancy Tuana, *The Less Noble Sex: Scientific, Religious, and Philosophical Conceptions of Woman's Nature* (Bloomington: Indiana University Press, 1993).

10. Cynthia Eagle Russett, *Sexual Science: The Victorian Construction of Womanhood* (Cambridge, MA: Harvard University Press, 1989).

11. Helen King, *Hippocrates' Woman: Reading the Female Body in Ancient Greece* (London: Routledge, 1998); and Lana Thompson, *The Wandering Womb: A Cultural History of Outrageous Beliefs About Women* (Amherst, NY: Prometheus Books, 1999).

12. Carroll Smith-Rosenberg and Charles Rosenberg, "The Female Animal: Medical and Biological Views of Women and Her Role in Nineteenth-Century America," *Journal of American History* 60 (September 1973): 333–34.

13. Carroll Smith-Rosenberg, "Puberty to Menopause: The Cycle of Femininity in Nineteenth-Century America," in Smith-Rosenberg, *Disorderly Conduct: Visions of Gender in Victorian America* (New York: Oxford University Press, 1985), p. 184.

14. Ann Wood, " 'The Fashionable Diseases': Women's Complaints and Their Treatment in Nineteenth-Century America," *Journal of Interdisciplinary History* 4, no. 9 (1973): 25–52.

15. John S. Haller and Robin M. Haller, *The Physician and Sexuality in Victorian America* (New York: W. W. Norton, 1974), p. 39.

16. Edward Clarke, *Sex in Education: A Fair Chance for Girls* (1874; repr., Salem, NH: Arno Press, 1972), pp. 126–27.

17. Martha H. Verbrugge, *Able-Bodied Womanhood: Personal Health and Social Change in Nineteenth-Century Boston* (New York: Oxford University Press, 1988).

18. James C. Whorton, *Nature Cures: The History of Alternative Medicine in America* (New York: Oxford University Press, 2002), p. 64; and James C. Whorton, "The First Holistic Revolution: Alternative Medicine in the Nineteenth Century," in *Examining Holistic Medicine*, ed. Douglas Stalker and Clark Glymour (Amherst, NY: Prometheus Books, 1985), pp. 37, 40.

19. Whorton, *Nature Cures*, p. 40.

20. Londa Schiebinger, *Nature's Body: Gender in the Making of Modern Science* (Boston: Beacon Press, 1993); Ludmilla Jordanova, *Sexual Visions: Images of Gender in Science and Medicine Between the Eighteenth and Nineteenth Centuries* (Madison: University of Wisconsin Press, 1989); and Cynthia Eagle Russett, *Sexual Science: The Victorian Construction of Womanhood* (Cambridge, MA: Harvard University Press, 1989). See also Carroll Smith-Rosenberg and Charles E. Rosenberg, "The Female Animal: Medical and Biological Views of Woman and Her Role in Nineteenth-Century America," *Journal of American History* 60 (September 1973): 332–56.

21. Susan E. Cayleff, *Wash and Be Healed: The Water-Cure Movement and Women's Health* (Philadelphia: Temple University Press, 1987): 53, 66, 74.

22. Jane B. Donegan, *"Hydropathic Highway to Health": Women and Water-Cure in Antebellum America* (Westport, CT: Greenwood Press, 1986), p. 194.

23. Naomi Rogers, "Women and Sectarian Medicine," in *Women, Health, and Medicine in America*, ed. Rima D. Apple (New Brunswick,

NJ: Rutgers University Press, 1990), pp. 273–302; and Thomas Neville Bonner, *To the Ends of the Earth: Women's Search for Education in Medicine* (Cambridge, MA: Harvard University Press, 1992).

24. Anne Taylor Kirschmann, "Adding Women to the Ranks, 1860–1890: A New View with a Homeopathic Lens," *Bulletin of the History of Medicine* 73, no. 3 (Fall 1999): 429–46; and Anne Taylor Kirschmann, "A Vital Force: Women Physicians and Patients in American Homeopathy, 1850–1930"(PhD diss., University of Rochester, 1999).

25. Edward H. Clarke, "Medical Education of Women," *Boston Medical and Surgical Journal* 81 (1869): 345–46.

26. Walter Channing, *Remarks on the Employment of Females as Practitioners in Midwifery, by a Physician* (Boston: Cummings and Hilliard, 1820), p. 7.

27. N. Williams, "A Dissertation on 'Female Physicians,'" *Boston Medical and Surgical Journal* 43 (1850): 69–75.

28. Mary Roth Walsh, *Doctors Wanted, No Women Need Apply: Sexual Barriers to the Medical Profession, 1835–1975* (New Haven, CT: Yale University Press, 1977), p. 135.

29. Dorothy M. Bernstein, "Women in Medicine: The Tortuous Path to Professionalism," *Minnesota Medicine* 75 (September 1992): 16–23.

30. Ephraim Fischoff, *Elizabeth Blackwell, First Woman M.D.*, Pearson Museum Monograph Series no. 81/4 (Springfield, IL: Southern Illinois University School of Medicine, Dept. of Medical Humanities, 1981).

31. John Harley Warner, "Science, Healing, and the Physician's Identity: A Problem of Professional Character in Nineteenth-Century America," in *Essays in the History of Therapeutics*, ed. W. F. Bynum and V. Nutton, special issue of *Clio Medica* 22 (1991): 66–77.

32. Linda Lehmann Goldstein, " 'Without Compromising in Any Particular': The Success of Medical Coeducation in Cleveland, 1850–1856," *Caduceus* 10 (1994): 101–15.

33. Virginia G. Drachman, *Hospital with a Heart: Women Doctors and the Paradox of Separatism at the New England Hospital, 1862–1969* (Ithaca, NY: Cornell University Press, 1984).

34. Steven J. Peitzman, *A New and Untried Course: Woman's Medical College and Medical College of Pennsylvania, 1850–1998* (New Brunswick, NJ: Rutgers University Press, 2000), p. 54.

35. Elizabeth Blackwell and Emily Blackwell, *Medicine as a Profession for Women* (New York: W. H. Tinson, 1860), pp. 9, 13.

36. Elizabeth Blackwell and Emily Blackwell, *Address on the Medical Education of Women* (New York: Baptist and Taylor, 1864).

37. Elizabeth Blackwell, "Letter to Ladies Desirous of Studying Medicine," *English Woman's Journal* 4, no. 23 (January 1860): 329–32.

38. Suellen Hoy, *Chasing Dirt: The American Pursuit of Cleanliness* (New York: Oxford University Press, 1995).

39. Fischoff, *Elizabeth Blackwell.*

40. Thomas Neville Bonner, *To the Ends of the Earth: Women's Search for Education in Medicine* (Cambridge, MA: Harvard University Press, 1992).

41. Regina Morantz-Sanchez, "Feminist Theory and Historical Practice: Rereading Elizabeth Blackwell," *History and Theory* 31, no. 4 (December 1992): 51–69.

42. Elizabeth Blackwell, "The Influence of Women in the Profession of Medicine" (Baltimore, 1890), pp. 8–9, 31.

43. Charles E. Rosenberg, "The Therapeutic Revolution: Medicine, Meaning, and Social Change in Nineteenth-Century America," *Perspectives in Biology and Medicine* 20 (1977): 485–506.

44. Elizabeth Blackwell, "Erroneous Method in Medical Education," *Essays in Medical Sociology* (London: Ernest Bell, 1902).

45. Regina Markell Morantz, "Feminism, Professionalism, and Germs: The Thought of Mary Putnam Jacobi and Elizabeth Blackwell," *American Quarterly* 34, no. 5 (Winter 1982): 459–78.

46. Louise Murphy Gearin, "The Giant Little Woman: Dr. Eliza-

beth Blackwell, The First Woman US Medical Graduate," *Journal of Medical Biography* 6 (1998): 89–96.

47. Elizabeth Blackwell, *Counsel to Parents: The Moral Education of Their Young Children in Relation to Sex under Medical and Social Aspects* (London: H. Smyth and Son, 1878).

48. Cathy Luchetti, *Medicine Women: The Story of Early-American Women Doctors* (New York: Crown, 1998).

49. Ellen S. More, *Restoring the Balance: Women Physicians and the Profession of Medicine, 1850–1995* (Cambridge, MA: Harvard University Press, 1995).

50. Mary Roth Walsh, *Doctors Wanted, No Women Need Apply*; and Regina Morantz-Sanchez, *Sympathy and Science: Women Physicians in American Medicine* (New York: Oxford University Press, 1985).

Pioneer Work in Opening the Medical Profession to Women

PREFACE

IT has often been urged that a record should be preserved of some of the first efforts by means of which the medical profession of our day has been opened to women.

In the belief that a large providential guidance may often be recognised in the comparatively trivial incidents of an individual life, this request of many friends is here complied with.

The possession of old journals and of family correspondence gives accuracy to these details of past years.

HASTINGS, 1895.

CONTENTS

CHAPTER I. EARLY YEARS

1821

Family Life in England—Walks around Bristol—May Missionary Meetings—A Vivid Reminiscence—Bristol Riots—Early Religious Impressions—Emigration to the United States—Schooldays in New York—Anti-slavery—Removal to Ohio—The Struggle of Life—Establishment of Boarding-school—The Wider Education of Women—Join the Episcopal Church—General Harrison's Election—Transcendentalism—The Rev. W. H. Channing's Congregation—Experiences in Henderson, Kentucky 51

CHAPTER II. EARNING MONEY FOR MEDICAL STUDY

1845

The Medical Idea taking Shape—Lack of an Absorbing Object—Objection to falling in Love—Struggles with Disinclination to the Study of Medicine—The Moral Aspect of the Work conquers—Resolution to earn Money for Study—Journey to Asheville, N.C.—Life in Asheville—Journey to Charleston, S.C.—Teaching at Mrs. du Pré's—Reading Medicine with Dr. S. H. Dickson—Sivori Concerts—Calhoun on States Rights—Dr. Warrington on Medical Study—Boarding-school Experiences—Summer at Aiken, S.C. 73

CHAPTER III. STUDY IN AMERICA

1847

Searching for a College—Application to Colleges of Philadelphia and New York—Interviews with Professors—Anatomical Study with Dr. Allen—Lectures at Dr. Warrington's—Application to other Schools—Joyful Result—Life at College—Residence in Blockley Almshouse—Graduation 101

CHAPTER IV. STUDY IN EUROPE

1849

Glimpse of the Black Country—Visit to Medical Institutions of Birmingham—Stay in London—Fashionable Life—Visits: to Dr. Carpenter, to Professor Owen, to St. Thomas's Hospital, to Dr. Wilkinson—Leave for Paris—Descriptive Letters—Interview with Lamartine—Interview with Police Official, with M. Louis—Difficulties to be overcome—Political Troubles in

Paris—Entrance into La Maternité—Severe Life there—Friendship with the *Interne*—A *Sortie* and Hypnotic *Séance*—Serious Accident—Visit to Gräfenberg—Life there—First Patient—Study in London—Admission to St. Bartholomew's—Visit to Rev. Dr. Leifchild—Hospital Experiences—Medical Scepticism awakens—Letter to Dr. S. H. Dickson—Social Relaxation—Woman's Rights Movement in the United States—Visit to Miss Nightingale—Visit to Lady Byron—Opening of the Great Exhibition—Anxious Discussion as to remaining in England—Farewell Visits—Last Days in England 135

CHAPTER V. PRACTICAL WORK IN AMERICA

1851

Settlement in New York—First Medical Consultation—Lectures on the Physical Education of Girls—Formation of Independent Dispensary—Quaker Help—Incorporation of the New York Infirmary, 1854—Letters descriptive of Early Difficulties—Purchase of House—Adoption of Child—First Drawing-room Address—Sister resolves to study—Letters to her whilst in Europe—Amusing Experience with Dr. Simpson of Edinburgh—Joined by Dr. Emily Blackwell in New York 219

CHAPTER VI. ENGLAND REVISITED

1858

Letter from Paris—Acquaintance with Dr. Trélat of La Salpêtrière—Addresses given in England—Result of London Addresses—Circular for proposed Hospital—Letters from London—Registered as English Physician, 1859—Reasons for returning to New York—Work there continued—Civil War—Ladies' Sanitary Aid Association established—Incidents of the War—Establishment of Infirmary Medical School—Letters from Miss Elizabeth Garrett—Sanitary Work of the New York Infirmary 239

CHAPTER VII. RETURN TO ENGLAND

1869

The Social Science Congress of 1869—Medical Work—Health Work—Moral Work 265

APPENDIX **277**

BIBLIOGRAPHY **287**

CHAPTER ONE

EARLY YEARS

1821

IT is a great advantage to have been born one of a large family group of healthy, active children, surrounded by wholesome influences.

The natural and healthy discipline which children exercise upon one another, the variety of tastes and talents, the cheerful companionship, even the rivalries, misunderstandings, and reconciliations where free play is given to natural disposition, under wise but not too rigid oversight, form an excellent discipline for after-life.

Being the third daughter in a family of nine brothers and sisters, who grew up to adult life with strong ties of natural affection, I enjoyed this advantage.

My earliest recollections are connected with the house in Bristol, No. 1 Wilson Street, near Portman Square, to which the family removed from Counterslip, where I was born, when I was about three years old. My childish remembrances are chiefly associated with my elder sisters, for being born between two baby brothers, who both died in infancy, I naturally followed my sisters' lead, and was allowed to be their playmate.

Our Wilson Street home had the advantage of possessing a garden behind it, containing fine trees; and also a large walled garden opposite to it, with fruit trees and many flowers and shrubs, which afforded us endless delight and helped to create an early love of Nature.

I cannot recall the sequel of incidents in this period of my life, for being so young when we moved to Wilson Street, the recollections of those early years are confused; but some things stand out, distinctly impressed on the memory.

My eldest sister had become possessed of a small telescope, and gazing through one of the garret windows, we thought we could spy the Duchess of Beaufort's woods over the tops of the houses. There was a parapet running along the front of the house, and we were seized with a desire for a more extensive view through the precious telescope than the garret window afforded, so a petition for liberty to go on to the roof was sent to papa in our names by my lively eldest sister. The disappointing answer soon came:

Anna, Bessie, and Polly, Your request is mere folly,
The leads are too high For those who can't fly.
If I let you go there, I suppose your next prayer
Will be for a hop To the chimney top!
So I charge you three misses, Not to show your phizes
On parapet wall, Or chimney so tall,
But to keep on the earth, The place of your birth.
"Even so," says papa. "Amen," says mama. "Be it so," says Aunt Bar.

The Aunt Barbara here referred to was a maiden sister of my father's, a somewhat stern though upright ruler of our youngest days; but the dear father, with his warm affection, his sense of fun, and his talent for rhyming, represented a beneficent Providence to me from my earliest recollection.

Another very vivid remembrance of that first period of childhood remains. My father was an active member of the "Independent" body, belonging to the Rev. Mr. Leifchild's Bridge Street congregation, and the May missionary meetings were a great event to us children, for, taking lunch with us, we sometimes picnicked in the gallery of the selected chapel, and divided our time between listening to thrilling stories of the missionaries and more physical pleasures. A number of these rather jolly divines often dined at our house, and the dinner party of the ministers was one of the incidents of the May meetings. There was a certain Mr. Burnet of Cork, who used to keep the table in a roar. To be allowed to dine and listen at a side-table was indeed a treat. But on one occasion, my name, alas! was in the Black Book, for some childish misdemeanour—I forget what; but the punishment I well remember. I was sent up to the attics, instead of being allowed to join the dinner party. Upstairs in the dark I leaned over the banisters, watched the light stream out from the dining-room as the servants carried the dishes in and out, and listened to the cheerful buzz of voices and frequent peals of laughter as the door opened. I felt very miserable, with also a sense of guilt that I should have been so wicked as to let my name get into the Black Book, for I always accepted, without thought of resistance, the decrees of my superiors. The fact that those in authority were capable of injustice or stupidity was a perception of later growth.

The impression made by this little incident on a childish mind was curiously shown on my revisiting Bristol, after an absence of nearly forty years. Wishing to see the scene of my early childhood, I called at the Wilson Street house, and its occupants kindly allowed me to enter my old home, the home which I remembered as so large, but which then looked so small. All was changed. The pleasant walled-in garden across the street, with its fine fruit trees, where we played for hours together with a neighbour's children, was turned into a carpenter's yard. The long garden behind the house, with its fine trees, and stable opening into a back street, was built over; but as I stood in the hall and looked up, I suddenly seemed to see a little childish face peeping wistfully over the banisters, and the whole scene of that dining-room paradise, from which the child was banished, rose vividly before me.

But a stranger incident still occurred as I stood there. The sound of a latch-key was heard in the hall-door, and a figure, that I at once recognised as my father's, in a white flannel suit, seemed to enter and look smilingly at me. It was only a momentary mental vision, but it was wonderfully vivid; and I then remembered what I had utterly forgotten—forgotten certainly for forty years—that our father would sometimes remain late at his sugar-house, and come home in the white flannel suit worn in the heated rooms of the refinery, letting himself into the house with a rather peculiar latch-key.

Far clearer and more varied recollections are, however, connected with the house in Nelson Street, to which we moved in 1824, and whence the family emigrated to New York in 1832.

This comfortable family home, made by throwing two houses together, with its walled-in courtyard leading to the sugar refinery and my father's offices, was our town residence for eight very happy years. Here the group of brothers and sisters grew up together, taking daily walks with our governess into the lovely environs of the then small town. We became familiar with St. Vincent's Rocks and the Hot Wells, with Clifton Down and Leigh Woods, which were not built on then. The Suspension Bridge across the Avon was a thing of the future, and Cook's Folly stood far away on the wild Durdham Down. In another direction, Mother Pugsley's field, with its healing spring, leading out of Kingsdown Parade, was a favourite walk—for passing down the fine avenue of elms we stood at the great iron gates of Sir Richard Vaughan's place, to admire the peacocks, and then passed up the lane towards Redland, where violets grew on the grassy banks and natural curiosities could be collected. All these neighbourhoods were delightfully free and open. Our governess encouraged our natural tastes, and the children's pennies were often expended in purchasing the landscape stones and Bristol diamonds offered for sale on Clifton Down. In still another direction, the "Brook," leading through pleasant fields to the distant Beaufort woods, had a never-ending charm. Daily, and often twice a day, the group of children with their governess wandered to these pleasant spots. In the summer time Weston-super-Mare and Clevedon gave endless seaside delights, and furnished a charming picture-gallery through all the subsequent wanderings of later life.

During the last years of our Bristol life, a house at Olveston, about nine miles from town, was rented as a summer residence. This afforded fresh delight. Not only was the neighbourhood beautiful, and interesting with views of the Welsh mountains seen across the Severn from a high common near by, and the remains of an old abbey where wolves' heads were formerly taken as tribute still remained; but the large, well-stocked garden was separated from the orchard by a rapid stream, over which two tiny bridges were thrown.

To active, imaginative children this little domain was a source of never-ending enjoyment, whether cherishing pet animals, cultivating gardens, or playing Robinson Crusoe. When not staying in town we lived in this pleasant place, my father driving out from business daily.

Only on rare occasions did any of the children go to school. Governesses and masters at home supplied the necessary book knowledge; and a passion for reading grew up, which made the present of a new book the greatest delight, and our own pocket-money was chiefly spent in buying books.

Whilst the home life was thus rich and satisfying to children, echoes from the outside world came vaguely to us. The Bristol Riots took place during this period, and I remember watching the glare of incendiary fires from the heights round our country home. Also I vividly recall the "chairing" of Bright and Protheroe, with their red and yellow colours, and the illumination of the house and premises in Nelson Street, in honour of this Liberal victory.

Our interest was early enlisted in the anti-slavery struggle then vigorously proceeding in England, and Wilberforce was an heroic name. The children voluntarily gave up the use of sugar, as a "slave product," although it was only in later years, when living in America, that they threw themselves ardently into the tremendous fight.

My father was an active member of the Independent body, and strongly opposed to the Established Church. "Rags of

Popery" was a phrase early learned in a parrot-like way. But a very strong sense of religion was early implanted. The Bible was held in affectionate reverence. Mrs. Sherwood's stories were favourite books; and although we soon learned to skip the endless disquisitions on metaphysical dogmas which they contained, yet goodness, gentleness, and reverence were inseparably blended with breezy commons, lovely woods, clear streams, and waterfalls, from reading those charming story-books. Religion thus became associated with all that was beautiful in Nature and lovely in social life.

Müller and Craik, the founders of the Plymouth Brethren, were then beginning their work in Bristol, and I was much impressed by the earnest eloquence of the young Scotch evangelist.

EMIGRATION TO THE UNITED STATES

The first eleven years of life had been passed under these happy influences of a healthy English home, when a great change of social surroundings took place, by my father's emigration to the United States with his large and increasing family.

Early life in America.—In the month of August 1832, the family party of eight children and seven adults sailed from Bristol in the merchant ship "Cosmo," reaching New York in about seven weeks.

The cholera was raging in England when we left; we found New York comparatively deserted, from the same cause, when we arrived, and several steerage passengers died during the voyage; but the family party remained in good health, and the ocean life furnished delightful experiences to the younger travellers.

The following six years were spent in New York and its suburb, Jersey City, across the bay.

As daily pupil in an excellent school in New York, entering ardently into the anti-slavery struggle, attending meetings and societies, the years passed rapidly away. Our brothers being younger than the three elder sisters, habits of unconscious independence amongst the sisters were formed, which became a matter of course.

Often in returning home from some evening meeting in New York the hourly ferry-boat would be missed, and we have crossed by the eleven or twelve o'clock boat, with no sense of risk or experience of annoyance.

We became acquainted with William Lloyd Garrison and other noble leaders in the long and arduous anti-slavery struggle. Garrison was a welcome guest in our home. He was very fond of children, and would delight them with long repetitions of Russian poetry.

But fierce antagonisms were already aroused by this bitter struggle; and on one occasion the Rev. Samuel H. Cox, a well-known Presbyterian clergyman, and his family, sought refuge at our country house. This gentleman had stated in the pulpit that the Lord Jesus belonged to a race with darker skins than ours. At once the rumour went abroad that "Dr. Cox had called Jesus Christ a nigger," and it was resolved forthwith to lynch him! So he came out to our country house on Long Island until the storm had blown over.

Removal to Ohio, 1838.—When I was seventeen years old my father removed from New York with his family to Cincinnati, then a small but flourishing town, on the Ohio River, where a promising opening for the extension of his business presented itself.

We left New York full of hope and eager anticipation. We were delighted with the magnificent scenery of the mountains and rivers as we crossed Pennsylvania by canal and stage (for it was before the time of railways), and sailed down the noble Ohio River, then lined with forests. With eager enjoyment of new scenes, the prosperous little Western town was reached. It was picturesquely situated on a plateau, overlooking the river, and surrounded by pleasant hills.

For a few months we enjoyed the strange incidents of early Western civilisation, so different from the older society of the East.

Amongst other curious experiences, we attended a public Fourth of July picnic, held in the neighbouring woods. At this festival, the well-known "Come-outers"[1]—the Wattles brothers—were the chief speakers. Augustus, the elder, had established in the unsettled districts of the West what he called "Humanity's Barn," where any human being might find a night's shelter. His younger brother, John, was a chief speaker on this special occasion, and he concluded his speech with the following (to us) astounding sentiment, which was loudly applauded by the large assembly present—viz.: "Priests, Lawyers, and Doctors, the Trinity of the Devil!"

But all these curious experiences were suddenly checked by a catastrophe which compelled us to face the stern realities of life, in the strange land to which we had just removed, without friends or pecuniary resources. This was the sudden death of our earthly Providence.

1. A term then applied in the West to those who were dissatisfied with every phase of our social life; they were generally noticeable for their long hair and peculiar mode of dressing.

The hot, oppressive summer of that Western climate proved too much for the English constitution of our father. Within a few months of our arrival in Cincinnati he died, after a short illness, from bilious fever, leaving his widow and nine children entirely unprovided for.

This irreparable loss completely altered our lives. Recovering from the first effects of the stunning blow, we began to realise our position, and the heavy responsibilities henceforth devolving on us. The three elder sisters set zealously to work, and in time established a day and boarding school for young ladies; whilst our eldest brother obtained a situation in the Court House of Cincinnati, under Major Gano.

For the next few years, until the younger children grew up and were able gradually to share in the work, we managed to support the family and maintain a home.

During this long struggle our minds rapidly opened to new views of social and religious duty in the untrammelled social atmosphere of the West.

The wider education of women was a subject then coming to the front; and we three sisters threw ourselves with ardour into the public conferences held in Cincinnati on this subject, actively supporting our staunch champion Lawyer Johnston, who ably opposed the reactionary efforts of the Roman Catholic Archbishop Purcell in his endeavour to check the liberal tendencies of the age in relation to women's education.

About this time we had joined the Episcopal Church, being confirmed by the venerable Bishop McIlvaine of Ohio. We became members of St. Paul's Church, of which the Rev. H.V. Johns was rector, entering heartily into its social life and teaching in its Sunday-school. We shared also in the stirring political contest which took place when General Harrison defeated Van Buren, the "Loco-foco"[2] candidate for the presidency. We attended political conventions and public meetings, and joined in singing political songs. It was a most exciting time.

Some years later, the New England Transcendental movement spread to the West. It was the era of the Brook Farm experiment. We became acquainted with the very intelligent circle of New England society settled in Cincinnati, of which the Rev. W. H. Channing was the attractive centre. This gentleman, nephew of Dr. Ellery Channing of Boston, and father of our present parliamentary representative of the Kettering Division of Northamptonshire, was afterwards well known in Liverpool and in London. He was a man of rare moral endowments and eloquence as a speaker. His social influence on a limited circle was remarkable. Men of thought and active intelligence gathered round him. Men from New England who were then intellectual leaders of Cincinnati thought—such as James Perkins, C. P. Cranch, William Greene, and Judge Walker—formed a society of which he was the inspiring centre, a society which strongly attracted us. The "Dial," and afterwards the "Harbinger," with its anticipation of social reorganisation, were then appearing. The writings of Cousin, Carlyle, and Fourier were keenly studied, and Emerson was revolutionising American thought. I well remember the glowing face with which I found Mr. Channing reading a book just received. "Sit down," he cried, "and listen to this!" and forthwith he poured forth extracts from Emerson's essays.

Notwithstanding our close and arduous teaching occupations, we eagerly shared in the active awakening of thought that

2. The popular name for the Democratic as opposed to the Republican candidate.

marked the time, and joined the Church of which Mr. Channing was minister.

In the year 1842, our elder brothers entering into business, the boarding-school was given up, and I occupied myself with private pupils. Whilst still engaged in this way I was invited to take charge of a girls' district school, to be established in the town of Henderson, situated in the western part of Kentucky. The invitation seemed to promise useful remunerative work, so it was accepted.

The region of Kentucky, where I then went, was a tobacco-growing district. I there gained my first practical experience of negro slavery and the crude civilisation of a Western slave State.

This being my first separation from the family, a constant correspondence was kept up with home. Some extracts from these letters will give a curious glimpse of Kentucky rural life fifty years ago.

Henderson: March 5, 1844.

No doubt you've reproached me for my silence, after promising to write the second day from my arrival, but we had a very long trip, and it was not till the morning of the fourth day that I set my foot in the mud of Henderson. The "Chieftain" left Cincinnati at two o'clock Wednesday morning, and in seven hours we made *twenty miles*. All seemed lazy on board the boat. The first night we laid up, on account of the fog; the second we spent at Louisville, the third at Evansville; we had on board a quantity of green wood, and stopped continually to take in fresh supplies. The captain, a fat, red-faced, good-natured fellow, went to sleep, or took matters very easily. As we entered the canal at Louisville he was standing on the hurricane-deck, at the head of the boat, apparently fast asleep; the helmsman steered immediately for the rough stone wall of the canal, and with a tremendous shock smashed in a great deal of the woodwork in the fore part of the boat. The captain gave one jump, wrung his hands, spun round, and went to sleep again. In the morning I went with Mr. S. into Louisville; there I got my watch-key mended (a providential piece of foresight, for 'twould have been impossible here), bought various little things, and saw also the famed Kentucky giant, and bade good-bye to Louisville, having been five hours passing through the canal. One afternoon Mr. S. was playing on his guitar on the side deck, when a great rough-looking boy made his appearance, and addressed me: "The ladies sent me to tell you to bring your man into the cabin, that he may sing for them." I translated for the *man's* benefit, and a good hearty laugh we had. One of Mr. S.'s favourite amusements was to stand on the hurricane-deck with me and joke about my *village*; every two or three dirty-looking shanties that we passed he would tell me to look out, for he had a presentiment that we were reaching Henderson. I grew almost nervous as we were approaching the situation, for really all the little towns we had passed looked so straggling, dingy, and uninteresting that it appeared to me almost impossible for a decent individual to inhabit them; you may imagine how I felt standing, for the last time, on a bright Saturday morning, with my last friend and remaining piece of civilisation, awaiting my destiny. The clerk approached. "Madam, we have reached Henderson"; the boat turns, I give one glance, three dirty old frame buildings, a steep bank covered with mud, some negroes and dirty white people at the foot, and behold all that I could see of my future home. I looked resolutely down, exclaiming (to my French friend), "Laide, vilain, horrible!" but the boat touched and I was hurried off. Upon my inquiring for Dr. Wilson, a rough-looking man presented his arm, three negroes seized my trunks, to "tote them up," the steamboat shoved off, and I followed my companion—holding his hand to prevent myself slipping down the bank. In the middle of the mud I stopped to see the last of our friend and civilisation; we waved our handkerchiefs till the boat was out of sight, and then, gulping down my tears and giving a few convulsive laughs, we proceeded on our way through a dirty, little, straggling, country village; we stopped before a small frame house, entered a low, shabbily-furnished room, where a poorly-dressed, sleepy-looking woman was introduced as Mrs. Wilson. I longed to be shown to my bedroom, for my head was in a perfect whirl, but I had to sit down and talk about I know not what. At last I ventured to request permission to go upstairs; the daughter showed me up old, crooked, creaking steps, and opened the bedroom door. How shall I describe it? A little window looking upon the side of a house not two yards from it, the rough board walls daubed with old whitewash, the bed, the furniture, dirty, covered with litter and dust, all gloomy and wretched. My disposition to cry vanished at once, tears froze far below zero; I smiled on my companion, who stood examining me, and asked to have my trunks carried up. This request brought my hostess, who with some confusion told me, "This was not to be my home, but that her niece was gone to make some preparations for my reception and would take me there in the evening, she being perfectly aware that I could not live in such a *hole*." The word "hole" revived me; the inhabitants of Henderson were, then, not perfectly blind; they had some little consciousness that there were degrees of decency; there was a small ray of comfort in that little word "hole." I descended, and soon found that everything proceeded with real Kentucky slowness. Begin to teach on Monday! This was utterly impossible! The idea seemed to them preposterous, the schoolhouse was hardly selected, the windows were broken, the floor and walls filthy, the plaster fallen off, the responsible trustees not appointed, the scholars unnotified of my arrival; no, 'twas impossible, I must wait a week; but the idea of spending an unnecessary week in Henderson was insupportable, so I urged and argued, and persuaded and ran about, till a man was sent to mend the windows, and another to clean the floor, and the Responsibles came to visit me, and promised to collect the scholars, and on Monday I was to begin. Then, to avoid the necessity of having to sit and repeat wearisome inanities, I set out, accompanied by the daughter, to view the so-called *city*. All looked dreary on a dull winter day—in fact, Henderson is a very small, very uninteresting country place, though, it must be confessed, the view of it from the river is the worst of all. Towards evening I took a look at my schoolhouse; nothing was done but mischief. The old negro had flooded the muddy floor with water and gone away, leaving the floor like the bed of the Nile; 'twas now too late to get the place into order. The people are very pious, nothing could be done Sunday; so, cursing the laziness of a slave society, I resigned myself to fate, and followed my young hostess—a tall, graceful, sleepy-eyed girl—to my new quarters.

A substantial, rough brick house opened its enormous gates to receive me. I entered a small, high-ceilinged bedroom, where I was to make one of *four*, and then my conductress glided away to bring her mother and two other sisters. The sight of the sisters somewhat consoled me, because I immediately hoped to be able to teach for my board. The mother received me with good-nature, and ever since I've been here the whole family have treated me with kindness to the extent of their knowledge, one portion of which is never to leave me alone, and I, who so love a hermit life for a good part of the day, find myself living in public, and almost losing my identity. Well, Sunday, and a refreshing Presbyterian sermon, of an eternity's duration, I must leave to your imagination. Monday I ran about, and at last seated myself in Dr. Wilson's parlour, where I received a visit from one of the Responsibles, a fussy, pompous little doctor, who talked *grandly*, whereupon I talked grandlier, upon which he told me this was an epoch in the history of Henderson. Then in came the other Responsibles, when I spoke and they rejoined, and the little doctor called to order, and after a wonderful quantity of fuss the schoolhouse was pitched upon, put into something like order, and on Tuesday morning I took my seat at the head of fourteen girls, and organised my school.

March 20, 1844.—So far as I can learn I give general satisfaction, but I believe the people are a little afraid of me, particularly when they see me read German (for I often forget myself with Hoffman). I am amused to learn accidentally how I have been talked over in every direction, and my teeth particularly admired in peculiarly Kentucky style. "Well, I do declare she's got a clean mouth, hasn't she!"—white teeth seeming remarkable where all use tobacco! All the chief people of the place have called on me, which plagues me dreadfully, as I have to return the calls, and find them in the lowest degree uninteresting, with nothing to do but knit, nothing to hear but their own petty affairs. Then they are most unmerciful in the length of visit. If they live in what is called out of town, nothing will satisfy but giving up the afternoon, taking tea, and sleeping. The sleeping I have victoriously fought against, but the rest I have sometimes been betrayed into, and have sat hour after hour striving dreadfully to take an interest in the gossip, swallowing yawns until my eyes watered, and then suddenly awaking out of a long reverie on all of you to the consciousness that everybody is sitting in an awkward silence, and that it is absolutely necessary to say something. The first evening I so spent I was rejoicing at the prospect of escape, for the watches had been pulled out, and it was declared late (half-past eight), when I was taken quite by surprise by seeing the Episcopal clergyman who was present seat himself by the table with a large Bible before him, wipe his spectacles, and give a preparatory hem! I gave an inward groan, sat down again and looked with a long face steadily at the fire, whilst a north-wester was blowing all the time through a crack of the door into my ear. As we knelt down, and I looked round at the funny kneeling figures and up at the walls of a real log cabin, and on one side at the immense wood fire, it all seemed so very odd that I almost began to doubt my own identity.

We have had miserable weather for more than a week. The house, though substantially built of brick, with a deep verandah all round, is dreadfully cold; the two immense brick-paved halls, which cross in the centre, have great doors almost always open. The four rooms occupying the four corners, in one of which we sleep, have chimneys, all of which smoke. Then none of the windows seem to fit, and there are holes in the wall where the plaster has been knocked off, and will be replaced, I suppose, next doomsday. 'Tis pretty much the same in the schoolhouse. There, one very cold day, I drew my feet on the bar of my chair, then I put on my worsted gloves, then drew on my blanket shawl; and, finally, finding a great blowing about my head from everywhere in general, I put on my hood! . . .

April 4.—The young ladies and gentlemen of Henderson are most contemptible walkers, opening wide their eyes at the idea of two or three miles, and telling doleful tales of blistered feet, wild bulls, and furious dogs, of which latter there is certainly a larger supply than at any place I have ever seen. Every negro has his pet dog, the more savage the better, and all the masters follow their example.

I had a good fright from some of them yesterday, as I was returning from school. I'd no sooner crossed the steps that lead into the lawn than an enormous brindled fellow, with black, devilish face, sprang furiously towards me, followed by two others, barking and showing their horrid jaws. Now, thought I, my time has come! I hesitated whether I should endeavour to tear their mouths open, or jump upon them and crush them, should the worst arrive. I involuntarily thought of A., who has a horror of dogs, and then called out in my blandest tones, "Poor fellows; po-or fellows!" The voice had the desired effect, and instead of having to fight Samson-wise, the gentlemen contented themselves with jumping upon me and knocking my dinner-tray out of my hand. I am in general quite a favourite with the canine race, and have not the slightest fear of them, which the ladies here can hardly believe, as their life is almost a torment to them for fear of dogs and cows; indeed, I would always sooner meet a dozen dogs than one negro, and the only uneasiness I have in taking my long, solitary walks proceeds from this; for of all brutes the human brute is the worst, and I never meet one in a lonely place without feeling a sudden perspiration.

I dislike slavery more and more everyday; I suppose I see it here in its mildest form, and since my residence here I have heard of no use being made of the whipping-post, nor any instance of downright cruelty. (It was really meant as an act of hospitality when they placed a little negro girl as a screen between me and the fire the other day!) But to live in the midst of beings degraded to the utmost in body and mind, drudging on from earliest morning to latest night, cuffed about by everyone, scolded at all day long, blamed unjustly, and without spirit enough to reply, with no consideration in any way for their feelings, with no hope for the future, smelling horribly, and as ugly as Satan—to live in their midst, utterly unable to help them, is to me dreadful, and what I would not do long for any consideration. Meanwhile I treat them civilly, and dispense with their services as much as possible, for which I believe the poor creatures despise me. The mistresses pique themselves on the advantageous situation of their blacks; they positively think them very well off, and triumphantly compare their position with that of the poor in England and other countries. I endeavour, in reply, to slide in a little truth through the small apertures of their minds, for were I to come out broadly with my simple, honest opinion I should shut them up tight, arm all their prejudices, and do ten times more harm than good. I do long to get hold of someone to whom I can talk frankly; this constant smiling and bowing and wearing a mask provokes me intolerably; it sends me internally to the other extreme, and I shall soon, I think, rush into the woods, vilify Henderson, curse the Whigs, and rail at the Orthodox, whose bells have been going in a fruitless effort at revivals ever since I have been here. Not, mind, mother, that I really have such diabolical feelings against the poor Orthodox in general and particular, but I have an intense longing to scream, and everyone here speaks in a whisper.

My school, I think I have told you, is limited to twenty-one; it has been full for some time, and many have been refused. The girls are a good, pleasant set, much more gentle than in Cincinnati, and all with faces that seem familiar to me; in fact, I have hardly seen a face in Henderson that does not torment me with a likeness to some former acquaintance. My school hours for the present are from nine to three. At half-past twelve I ring my bell, when there is a general rush and devouring. I uncover the tin knife-box devoted to me, and find regularly inside a saucer with three or four little slices of ham, a roll, a piece of corn bread, a cup of cream, and a raw egg; the latter I throw into the hot ashes, and when it has split with a loud report I take it out, and, peeling off the coating of burnt egg and ashes, am generally happy enough to find a little clean piece in the middle, which I swallow, and burn my throat. Then I put on my hood and gloves, and walk up and down under a tree in front of the schoolhouse, eating the remainder, and endeavouring not to think of you all, as I find it does not assist the digestion.

I used to look sentimentally to one corner of the heavens and fancy I saw you all, when one evening, to my amazement, I beheld the sun set in that corner, so I had to turn right round and look in the opposite direction, anathematising the river for being so stupid as to wind, and convert the sublime imaginings of a forlorn damsel into a ridiculous blunder.

I have at present four music scholars, and one out-of-school French, but two go for boarding. I teach ten hours, three days of the week, and wish the other three were similarly filled; but it is small remuneration for such an outlay of breath, and as soon as I have the opportunity I shall fly off to some other point of the compass, where at any rate I may learn myself while teaching others. Carlyle's name has never even been distantly echoed here, Emerson is a perfect stranger, and Channing, I presume, would produce a universal fainting-fit.

Henderson.

I was delighted to receive my box last Sunday, the 12th; the things do admirably, the dresses I like exceedingly, they are both very pretty.

The people here begin to interest me more than they did at first; all continue very kind, and I think well satisfied. When I came here, I did not care one straw what was thought of my personal appearance, I dressed entirely from a principle of self-respect; now I sometimes dress for others, and feel a slight satisfaction if the glass tells me I shall not scare people. Is not this a good sign? . . . Do not imagine I am going to make myself a whole just at present; the fact is I cannot find my other half here, but only about a sixth, which would not do. There are two rather eligible young males here, whose mothers have for some time been electioneering for wives; one tall, the other short, with very pretty names, of good family, and with tolerable fortune, but unfortunately one seems to me a dolt, the other, well, not wise, so I keep them at a respectful distance, which you know I am quite capable of doing.

There is a spot called Lovers' Grove, about three-quarters of a mile from the town, a sweet place on the river bank, encircled by trees, with a hill behind, and a delightful walk by the river-side connecting it with the "city." This used to be my Sunday afternoon stroll, but unfortunately it is the favourite resort of the beaux and belles of Henderson, who, during the summer, after afternoon church, regularly promenade thither, in groups of four or five, and meet accidentally on purpose. Here they stroll about, recline on the grass, watch the steamboats, flirt a very little (it being Sunday), and carve one another's names, and sentimental verses, on the unfortunate locust trees. I had many offers of an escort thither and as many beaux as I might desire. I went once or twice, but at last got dreadfully tired of it, so while my party was busily engaged round a tree, I started off on a good brisk walk home, where, some time after, the others arrived, in some consternation to know how or why I had so suddenly vanished. I laughed at them and their sentimental doings, and they have not invited me since.

I had a very pleasant drive yesterday to make a bridal call on the Presbyterian minister, who has been quite polite. The country reminded me in some parts of our charming Staten Island drives, though the scenery here will not, of course, compare with that little gem.

The people of Henderson were all very friendly to me personally, and my relations always pleasant with them; but the injustice of the state of society made a gradually deepening impression on my mind. The inhabitants lived in constant fear of an outbreak among the slaves. Women did not dare to walk in the pleasant woods and country around the village, for terror of runaway slaves. Painful social contrasts constantly forced themselves on my notice. I well remember sitting with my hostess, who was reclining in her rocking-chair, on the broad, shaded verandah, one pleasant Sunday morning, listening to the distant church bells and the rustling of the locust trees, when the eldest daughter, a tall, graceful girl, dressed for Sunday, in fresh and floating summer drapery, came into the verandah on her way to church. Just at that moment a shabby, forlorn-looking negro in dirty rags approached the verandah; he was one of the slaves working in the tobacco plantation. His errand was to beg the mistress to let him have a clean shirt on that Sunday morning. The contrast of the two figures, the young lady and the slave, and the sharp reprimand with which his mistress from her rocking-chair drove the slave away, left a profound impression on my mind. Kind as the people were to me personally, the sense of justice was continually outraged; and at the end of the first term of engagement I resigned the situation.

Chapter Two

Earning Money for Medical Study

1845–1847

T*he idea taking shape.*—When I returned from the Kentucky engagement the family had removed to the pleasant suburb of Walnut Hills, where the well-known Lane Theological Seminary, under the direction of the Beechers and Professor Stowe, was situated. This healthy place, with its intellectual resources, became the home for many years. I found the family sharing a delightful house with the Rev. Mr. and Mrs. Vail, to whom it belonged, who, with their charming daughter and the professor and elder students of the seminary, formed a very intelligent society.

It was during the residence of the family on Walnut Hills that the noble-hearted woman, Lucy Stone, became the wife of an elder brother of mine.

My brothers were engaged in business, my sisters variously occupied, the family life was full and active, and for a while I keenly enjoyed the return home. But I soon felt the want of a more engrossing pursuit than the study of music, German, and metaphysics, and the ordinary interests that social life presented.

It was at this time that the suggestion of studying medicine was first presented to me, by a lady friend. This friend finally died of a painful disease, the delicate nature of which made the methods of treatment a constant suffering to her. She once said to me: "You are fond of study, have health and leisure; why not study medicine? If I could have been treated by a lady doctor, my worst sufferings would have been spared me." But I at once repudiated the suggestion as an impossible one, saying that I hated everything connected with the body, and could not bear the sight of a medical book.

This was so true, that I had been always foolishly ashamed of any form of illness. When attacked many years before by intermittent fever, I desperately tried to walk off the deadly chill; and when unable to do so, shut myself up alone in a dark room till the stage of fever was over, with a feeling that such subjection to disease was contemptible. As a school-girl I had tried to harden the body by sleeping on the floor at night, and even passing a couple of days without food, with the foolish notion of thus subduing one's physical nature. I had been horrified also during my schooldays by seeing a bullock's eye resting on its cushion of rather bloody fat, by means of which one of the professors wished to interest his class in the wonderful structure of the eye. Physiology, thus taught, became extremely distasteful to me. My favourite studies were history and metaphysics, and the very thought of dwelling on the physical structure of the body and its various ailments filled me with disgust.

So I resolutely tried for weeks to put the idea suggested by my friend away; but it constantly recurred to me.

Other circumstances forced upon me the necessity of devoting myself to some absorbing occupation. I became impatient of the disturbing influence exercised by the other sex. I had always been extremely susceptible to this influence. I never remember the time from my first adoration, at seven years old, of a little boy with rosy cheeks and flaxen curls when I had not suffered more or less from the common malady—falling in love. But whenever I became sufficiently intimate with any individual to be able to realise what a life association might mean, I shrank from the prospect, disappointed or repelled.

I find in my journal of that time the following sentence, written during an acute attack:—

> I felt more determined than ever to become a physician, and thus place a strong barrier between me and all ordinary marriage. I must have something to engross my thoughts, some object in life which will fill this vacuum and prevent this sad wearing away of the heart.

But the struggle with natural repugnance to the medical line of life was so strong that I hesitated to pass the Rubicon, and fought many a severe battle with myself on the subject.

At this time I had not the slightest idea of how to become a physician, or of the course of study necessary for this purpose. As the idea seemed to gain force, however, I wrote to and consulted with several physicians, known to my family, in various parts of the country, as to the possibility of a lady becoming a doctor.

The answers I received were curiously unanimous. They all replied to the effect that the idea was a good one, but that it was impossible to accomplish it; that there was no way of obtaining such an education for a woman; that the education required was long and expensive; that there were innumerable obstacles in the way of such a course; and that, in short, the idea, though a valuable one, was impossible of execution.

This verdict, however, no matter from how great an authority, was rather an encouragement than otherwise to a young and active person who needed an absorbing occupation.

If an idea, I reasoned, were really a valuable one, there must be some way of realising it. The idea of winning a doctor's degree gradually assumed the aspect of a great moral struggle, and the moral fight possessed immense attraction for me.

This moral aspect of the subject was increased by a circumstance which made a very strong impression on me. There was at that time a certain Madame Restell flourishing in New York. This person was a noted abortionist, and known all over the country. She was a woman of great ability, and defended her course in the public papers. She made a large fortune, drove a fine carriage, had a pew in a fashionable church, and though often arrested, was always bailed out by her patrons. She was known distinctively as a "female physician," a term exclusively applied at that time to those women who carried on her vile occupation.

Now, I had always felt a great reverence for maternity—the mighty creative power which more than any other human faculty seemed to bring womanhood nearer the Divine.

The first serious essay I ever attempted was on "The Motherhood of the Race, or Spiritual Maternity"—that great fact of universal love and service which is the formative principle striving to express itself in the lower physical manifestations.

The gross perversion and destruction of motherhood by the

abortionist filled me with indignation, and awakened active antagonism. That the honourable term "female physician" should be exclusively applied to those women who carried on this shocking trade seemed to me a horror. It was an utter degradation of what might and should become a noble position for women.

Being at that time a reader of Swedenborg, and strongly impressed by his vivid representations of the unseen world, I finally determined to do what I could to "redeem the hells," and especially the one form of hell thus forced upon my notice.

My journals of those days, 1845, are full of the various difficulties encountered as this determination took root.

I find it written:—

Doctor Muzzey (a well-known Cincinnati doctor) was horrified at the idea of a woman's going to the Parisian schools, which he visited some years ago; and he declares that the method of instruction was such that no American or English lady could stay there six weeks.

Mrs. Beecher Stowe thought, after conversation with Professor Stowe, that my idea was impracticable, though she confessed, after some talk, that if carried out it might be highly useful. She also spoke of the strong prejudice which would exist, which I must either crush or be crushed by. I felt a little disappointed at her judgment and the hopelessness of all help from Dr. M. I resolved to write to Dr. Cox (our family physician when we lived in the East), as a last hope for the present.

Sunday, May 4.—I read my letter to Dr. Cox to Mrs. Vail, who sympathises strongly with my desire. She stated Dr. Peck's opinion of the impossibility of a lady studying in Paris, but asserts that the most thorough education can be obtained in private. I will not, however, make up my mind too hastily on so important a subject.

Wednesday, 14*th.*—I mentioned my plan to Mr. Perkins. He talked it over a little, and then said with a bright face: "I do wish you would take the matter up, if you have the courage—and you have courage, I know." So invigorating was his judgment, that I felt at the moment as if I could conquer the world. He offered with real interest to obtain the opinion of the Boston physicians, to talk with Dr. Avery, and lent me a book of Jackson's Memoirs which gives much information relative to the French schools.

But a little later it is written:—

I felt cold and gloomy all day; read in Jackson's Memoirs, and felt almost disheartened at the immensity of the field before me. I hesitate as if I were about to take the veil, but I am gradually coming up to the resolution.

Again it is written:—

I heard an admirable sermon from Mr. Giles, an English minister, on Christian worship; very logical, full of poetry, some of the sentences so perfect that I held my breath till they were finished. I thought much on my future course, and turned for aid to that Friend with whom I am beginning to hold true communion. It cannot be my fancy, Jesus Christ must be a living Spirit, and have the power of communicating with us, for one thought towards Him dispels all evil, and earnest, continued thought produces peace unspeakable.

May 20.—Harry brought me home last evening a letter from Dr. Cox; my hand trembled as I took it. It was kind, giving the necessary information, but perfectly non-committal as to advice. I carried the letter over this morning to the lady friend who had promised to help me pecuniarily. I made up my mind fully to undertake the study if she fulfilled her promise, and already I felt separated from the rest of womankind; I trembled and hoped together. But alas for promises and plans; she offered to lend me 100 dollars—when I am told that I shall want 3,000 dollars! I did not express my disappointment, but asked who would be likely to assist further? She did not know, but thought the plan I had suggested of teaching, and laying up money for a few years, decidedly the best.

Thrown thus entirely on my own resources, I finally resolved to accept a teacher's position in a school in North Carolina, where, whilst accumulating money for future use, I could also commence a trial of medical study, for the Rev. John Dickson, who was principal of the school, had previously been a doctor.

My old diary of those years, still existent, vividly portrays the anxiety and painful effort with which I left the family circle and ordinary social life, and took the first step in my future medical career. I felt that I was severing the usual ties of life, and preparing to act against my strongest natural inclinations. But a force stronger than myself then and afterwards seemed to lead me on; a purpose was before me which I must inevitably seek to accomplish.

My own family showed the warmest sympathy with my plans. It was before the time of railways; the roads through Kentucky were little travelled; several rivers had to be forded, and three lines of mountains to be crossed. Two of my brothers determined to drive me to my unknown destination amongst the mountains of North Carolina. So the carriage was packed with books and comforts for the eleven days' journey, and on June 16, 1845, with loving good-byes and some tears, in spite of strong efforts to restrain them, I left home for Asheville, North Carolina, to begin preparation for my unknown career.

I find interesting details of that long drive, when every day took me farther and farther away from all that I loved. We forded more than one rapid river, and climbed several chains of the Alleghanies in crossing through Kentucky and Tennessee into North Carolina. The wonderful view from the Gap of Clinch Mountain, looking down upon an ocean of mountain ridges spread out endlessly below us, and seen in the fresh light of an early morning, remains to this day as a wonderful panorama in memory.

We at last reached our destination—viz. the school and parsonage of the Rev. John Dickson (formerly a physician), where I was to teach music. The situation of Asheville, entirely surrounded by the Alleghanies, was a beautiful plateau, through which the rapid French Broad River ran.

I must here note down an experience occurring at that time, unique in my life, but which is still as real and vivid to me as when it occurred.

I had been kindly welcomed to my strange new home, but the shadow of parting with the last links to the old life was upon me. The time of parting came. My two brothers were to leave on their return journey early on the following morning. Very sadly at night we had said farewell. I retired to my bedroom and gazed from the open window long and mournfully at the dim mountain outlines visible in the starlight—mountains which seemed to shut me away hopelessly from all I cared for. Doubt and dread of what might be before me gathered in my mind. I was overwhelmed with sudden terror of what I was undertaking. In an agony of mental despair I cried out, "Oh God, help me, support me! Lord Jesus, guide, enlighten me!" My very being went out in this yearning cry for Divine help. Suddenly, overwhelmingly, an answer came. A glorious presence, as of brilliant light, flooded my soul. There was nothing visible to the physical sense; but a spiritual influence so joyful, gentle, but powerful, surrounded me that the despair which had overwhelmed me vanished. All doubt as to the future, all hesitation as to the rightfulness of my purpose, left me, and never in after-life returned. I *knew* that, however insignificant my individual effort might be, it was in a right direction, and in accordance with the great providential ordering of our race's progress.

This is the most direct personal communication from the Unseen that I have ever consciously had; but to me it is a revealed experience of Truth, a direct vision of the great reality of spiritual existence, as irresistible as it is incommunicable.

During my few months' stay in this friendly household I borrowed medical books from the Doctor's library, for my purpose of becoming a physician was known and approved of.

On one occasion a fellow-teacher laughingly came to me with a dead cockchafer, which had been smothered between her pocket-handkerchiefs, and offered it to me as a first subject for dissection. I accepted the offer, placed the insect in a shell, held it with a hair-pin, and then tried with my mother-of-pearl-handled penknife to cut it open. But the effort to do this was so repugnant that it was some time before I could compel myself to make the necessary incision, which revealed only a little yellowish dust inside. The battle then fought, however, was a useful one. In my later anatomical studies I never had so serious a repugnance to contend with.

The winter passed pleasantly away in beautiful Asheville. I was in friendly relations with all around me. In my leisure time I studied in the pleasant grove which connected the school with the church, rejoicing in the ever-changing mountain outline visible through the trees. The "Harbinger," with its bright visions of associated life, came regularly to me, and nurtured that faith in co-operation as the necessary future of society which has become one of my articles of faith, my chief regret at this time being the stoppage of my attempt to teach coloured children to read, as this was forbidden by the laws of North Carolina!

The following letters describe the life in North Carolina:—

Asheville: June 29, 1845.

DEAR M.,—My first impressions of Asheville are decidedly pleasant. I find the Rev. Mr. D. a well-educated, intelligent man, beloved by all, and regarded quite as a father by all his pupils. He reminds me continually of Mr. L. in the shortness of his legs and the activity of mind and body, in superficiality of thought, and obliging social disposition. Mrs. D. is decidedly lovable, quite a little lady, ever cheerful, kind, and intelligent, performing her numerous duties like a small, true Christian. . . .

Asheville: 1845.

DEAR H.,—I am very glad to find that you have the feelings of a gentleman, that though you would not promise to write to me, you perform, which is decidedly the better of the two. Now I have to call you and S. to account for your breach of promise. What is the reason you did not come to my window, as you agreed to do, the morning you left Asheville? I got up before four o'clock and waited and watched, at last grew angry, and wished in revenge that you might have fine weather and plenty of ripe blackberries the whole way! It was a very shabby trick, and if you do not render a satisfactory explanation I shall—scold you well when next we meet.

Your domestic items all interest me. How do you like the change of teachers in the school, and who will superintend your room? Will Dr. Ray still teach? You must tell me also what day school begins, that I may think of you and Billy sitting with grave faces behind the little wooden desks, rivalling one another in intense application.

Did you take home any stones for our cabinets? Does the collecting fit continue, or has it vanished with the departure of Mr. Hildreth? I have not obtained many specimens as yet; little Sarah Dickson takes great interest in bringing me what she considers pretty rocks, and putting them on a newspaper on my window seat. I was really surprised the other day to see how pretty they looked, though, of course, not of much value—little bits of quartz, white, grey, brown, pink; a stone full of mica, which looks like a piece of lead ore; a conglomerate of gneiss quartz tinged with some metallic substances, and with garnets embedded in some of the stones; and flints of various colours; nothing to a professed mineralogist, but pleasing to me.

Last week I went to a party at Mrs. P.'s. She has a separate establishment from the hotel, with which she does not choose to have anything to do. I was invited to meet some Charleston ladies who had called on me, and made themselves very agreeable. I suppose you would have been most pleased with the eatables (the ice-cream, whips, jelly, and cakes were delicious), but what delighted me was a little Channing glorification (M. will understand what I mean) that Mrs. Carr (the lady who so resembles Ellen Channing) and I held in the garden. She has never seen our Mr. Channing, but the Doctor used to visit at their house, and she described with enthusiasm a splendid sermon that she heard him deliver in Philadelphia. I replied by describing the eloquence of our Mr. C. Then she expatiated on the kindness and loveliness of the Doctor's character, to which I added a description of the goodness, purity, and the angelicalness of his nephew; whereupon she expressed a great desire to see him, and I said that I should consider it one of the greatest of blessings to have enjoyed the social intercourse of the good Doctor. The conversation was quite a treat to me—a sort of safety-valve to heterodox steam that I lacked so deplorably at Henderson.

My playing seemed to give satisfaction; the piano is a beautiful one, like ours on a more brilliant scale, and as there was no one to rival me in the instrumental way I raised the top, played the "Pot Pourri," and made a tremendous noise. (I do wish that minister would stop singing his nasal hymn-tunes just underneath me; he has been at it all day, and it quite puts me out.)

I also showed some tricks which puzzled the company—particularly a very tall man, with long, projecting nose and retreating forehead, who looked like a stupid fox. Miss Jane P. was seated in a corner, behind a little table, on which were draughts arranged as the nuns of the Lady Abbess, she challenging everybody to introduce the four cavaliers unknown to the blind mistress. Everybody said it was not possible, and Miss Jane turned triumphantly to me to know if I could do it. I said I could not only introduce the four knights, but their four squires also, and then suffer knights, squires, and four nuns to elope, without the blind Abbess having the slightest suspicion of the defection. Everybody thought it impossible, but when I actually performed the feat they looked upon me as half a conjuror—particularly the stranger fox—and Mrs. Dickson thought it was hardly safe that I should occupy the front bedroom in a young ladies' boarding-school. I also amused them with the three jealous couples crossing the stream; we were all very merry, and I did more talking than I have accomplished in the same space of time for many a day. On our return home, the young gentleman who accompanied me said that if he had only known I was coming he would have gone from New York to Cincinnati, to escort me to Asheville (I did not tell him how very glad I was he did not know it); and on my expressing a wish to visit Mount Pisgah, he assured me that to the very next party that was made up he would be sure to see that I received an invitation. (I did not say he need not trouble himself, that I should get the invitation without his interference; I only thought all that, for I am growing very polite in my *manners*.)

. . . About a week ago I rode to the Sulphur Springs, which are about four miles from Asheville; they are not much resorted to, the country round being tangled and rather uninteresting. The springs, however, are situated in a delightful valley, through which the wind blew most refreshingly; a roofed platform is erected in the midst of the grass plat, the perfectly clear water welling up into a marble basin on one side, and then flowing away in a little rivulet. I found a country woman resting herself on the platform, with a bright, pleasant face and very communicative. I sat and talked to her and thought of the woman of Samaria; presently a bilious-looking Southerner came down and drank a dipper full of water, which dispelled all the illusion, for my imagination conjured up rice-swamps and clanking chains.

I have not taken many walks about here, for the weather, though delightful for July, is too hot for walking, and riding seems out of the question, it being harder to get a horse here even than it was at Henderson. Dr. Dickson has one old fellow, but he is used in the fields a good deal, and one person cannot ride alone. Borrowing or hiring seems equally impossible, so I shall be the poorest rider in the family apparently, for I suppose Henry's "nice little pony," and our three (?) other horses, will be kept in constant use.

I find it equally impossible to get a partner in chess; Dr. Dickson understands no such games, and disapproves of them, so I cannot train any of the girls, and Miss C. does not care to play. I set up the men one afternoon and tried to beat myself; but it would not do, I could get up no enthusiasm, so I put the pieces away in despair, and used the board as a writing-desk.

Tell me all the home news: what M. does and Ellen and Kate, what nonsense H. talks and S.'s puns, the visits they receive and the excursions they make.

If you hear of any new books let me know, for I imagine they do not find their way up here very quickly. I have Littel's "Living Age" regularly, and I am reading Alison's "History of Europe"; but such a thing as a novel Dr. Dickson reprobates, and all he calls light reading.

Now, Howy, do you not think I am very good to send you such a long letter for your little scrap? Write me a full sheet soon.

Asheville: July 27, 1845.

DEAR MOTHER,—I received your welcome letter last night while engaged in your favourite Saturday evening's employment—singing hymns. A stranger minister who was to preach next day had just arrived, and I, seated at the piano, surrounded by the girls, was supplying him with sacred entertainment, when Howard Dickson laid your letter beside me. I smiled, and gave an involuntary quaver in the "Come, Holy Spi—," which made the girls giggle; but seeing the four eyes of the two ministers bent astonishedly upon us, I pulled a long face, the girls straightened theirs, and we continued—"rit, heavenly Dove."

I soon ran off with a candle and my letter, and read with eagerness all the profane parts, and most of the religious, as it is a first letter. I am very glad that you derive so much peaceful satisfaction from Upham. I know it has a soothing influence, for whenever I had to go into your room of an afternoon I found you asleep on the bed with the book in your hand; but I find no lack of such books here—Jonathan Edwards on the Affections, which I have lately read, has the same peaceful tendency.

I have just performed my first professional cure, and am already dubbed Dr. Blackwell by the household. I mesmerised away a severe headache that afflicted Miss O'Heara, a kind-hearted, child-like, black-haired little old maid, the favourite of the family and especial pet of the children. She had just recovered from a very severe attack of illness, and great suffering in the mouth from calomel, which made her declare that no physician ought to receive his diploma till he has been salivated, that he may know the torture he is inflicting on his patients. I went into her room last night, and found her suffering from an intense throbbing headache. I offered to relieve her, half doubting my own powers, never having attempted anything of the kind; but in a quarter or half an hour she was entirely relieved, and declared some good angel had sent me to her aid.

I have just returned from the Sunday-school which we have organised to-day for the slaves. When I first came here I determined to teach all the slaves I could to read and write, and elevate them in every way in my power, as the only way I could reconcile it to my conscience to live amongst them; but to my consternation I found that the laws forbade it, and that Dr. Dickson was not willing to evade them. Not the slightest effort was made to instruct them in any way, except that now and then a sermon was preached to them; but they had to labour on without a ray of light or hope. It was intolerable to me, and I proposed at last we should have Sunday-school, and give them real instruction; and as such a scheme had been talked of about a year ago, I found a few who were willing to engage in the undertaking. Accordingly, this afternoon at three o'clock we made a beginning—four ladies and one gentleman, with about twenty-five scholars; we have a class of men, women, boys, and two of girls. I take one of the latter, four girls, from eight to twelve years old. I assure you I felt a little odd, sitting down before those degraded little beings, to teach them a religion which the owners professed to follow whilst violating its very first principles, and audaciously presuming to stand between them and the Almighty. As I looked round the little room and saw those ladies holding forth to their slaves, fancying that now they were fulfilling every duty and were quite model mistresses, I longed to jump up, and, taking the chains from those injured, unmanned men, fasten them on their tyrants till they learned in dismal wretchedness the bitterness of that bondage they inflict on their brethren. But one person can do nothing. I sat quietly teaching, and reserved my indignation to vent on this inoffensive white paper. I am afraid much cannot be done for the slaves in this way; their minds are so obscured, and oral instruction is so tedious, that the patience of both teachers and scholars may be worn out. I, however, shall do my utmost to illuminate both head and heart, and the poor children thanked me with humble sincerity this afternoon for my efforts.

You need not be afraid I shall make myself conspicuous, or gain the hated name of Abolitionist. I sometimes reproach myself for my prudence and the calmness with which I answer some outrageous injustice, while I am really raging with indignation; but it is the only way in which I can hope to do any good, for the slightest display of feeling arms all their prejudices, and I am no orator to convert by a burst of passionate eloquence; so I must even go on in my own quiet manner, knowing that it does not proceed from cowardice.

I wish I could give you a cheering account of numerous music scholars and French and German classes, but the place is too small for anything of the sort. I hear constantly a great deal about Charleston; everybody seems connected with that city, and a great many of the inhabitants are spending the summer here and at the Springs. I mean to make some inquiries about the schools and teachers of that city; it would be a pleasant residence in some respects. I mention this, not from any serious idea of going there, but that you may know the schemes that are passing through my mind. I am fixed here till December.

My brain is as busy as can be, and consequently I am happy; for one is only miserable when stupid and lazy, wasting the time and doing no good to self or anybody else.

So you, too, mother, confirm Henry's account of the "fine doings" on our quiet Walnut Hills. I shall really begin to think that I have been the evil genius of the place, withholding the rain from the garden, the visitors from the house; for no sooner am I gone than floods of both flow down and up, and everywhere are greenness and gaiety. Very well; I certainly won't come back to bring a blight into Paradise. . . . But, seriously, if Miss A. G. comes up, I hope M. will consider it a call and return it with dignity, for it seems to me H. is growing wild and turning our house into a sort of banqueting-hall for Comus and his crew, which I beg M. to set her face against by taking every visit to herself. . . .

My white bonnet is much admired here. Miss Charlotte Carr sent to borrow it the other day, and has made one its exact image, flowers and all. I felt quite proud in setting the fashion in Asheville!

In 1846 the Asheville school was broken up, and I resolved to try my fortunes in the South, journeying with Mrs. John Dickson to Charleston, S.C., exchanging the fine mountain country for the level rice-fields of South Carolina. It was a striking journey—a transformation scene! It is thus described in a journal of that date:—

On January 14 we left by stage early in the morning. We jolted off in the bright moonlight; the ground was frozen hard and very rough. I walked with Flinn over the Blue Ridge and the Saluda, another branch of the Alleghanies. The weather was beautiful, the air invigorating, and the mountain seemed to deserve its name. On the top of the Saluda a stone marks the boundary of the two Carolinas. I hesitated at crossing it, for my affections are all with the "old North State." At the foot we drank to its health from the Poinsett Spring, as we had promised John to do. A little afterwards we passed the wildest scenery I ever remember to have seen. The road wound down the south side of the mountain in very abrupt curves, so as to form a succession of terraces one above the other; whilst, on the opposite side, the wooded mountain ridge, though so near, was softened by mist, and seemed to tower to tremendous heights, though I was surprised to see how this height seemed to lessen as we descended. We reached Greenville late, after eighty miles of horribly rough staging; there we spent the next day, and I took a pleasant walk with Flinn by the reedy river, which rushes in cascades through rocks and wooded hills. The next two days we travelled through pretty, undulating country, gradually becoming more level. I saw the first characteristic swamp, also the palmetto and the strange grey moss, a yard long, hanging from the trees. We spent a night in Columbia. It seemed a strange revival of old associations to enter a city once more. The hotel was full of horse-racers engaged in betting. The next day a rapid railway journey brought us to Charleston by two o'clock. The country between Columbia and Charleston was much prettier than I expected. The lovely day made everything beautiful; the numerous pines, the holly, wild orange, live oak, and other evergreens seemed to give the lie to January. The moss, hanging one or two yards long from the trees, looked like gigantic webs or the ghosts of weeping willows; the rice-fields, under water, were as blue as the sky; the level cotton-fields, extending for hundreds of acres, with their belts of evergreens, were strange and beautiful.

When we reached Charleston we were met at the station by Dr. Sam. Dickson's carriage, with its very gentlemanly negro coachman, who had been sent for Flinn and "the lady." So I said good-bye to kind Mrs. John Dickson, and, driving softly along to a large old-fashioned house, surrounded by a garden full of tall evergreens, I entered a spacious hall and was welcomed by Dr. Sam. and Mrs. Dickson and their eldest daughter, and ushered into a handsome drawing-room, cloak, hood, smoke, and all.

Dr. Samuel H. Dickson, who thus hospitably welcomed me, was a distinguished physician of Charleston and professor in the Medical College of that town. He gave me kind encouragement in relation to my medical studies. Through his influence I soon obtained a position as teacher of music in the fashionable boarding-school of Mrs. DuPré (a connection of the Doctor), where I taught for some hours every day, spending all my spare time in pursuing the medical studies which Dr. Dickson directed. Every morning a couple of hours were devoted before breakfast to learning the necessary rudiments of Greek (for I had only so far been acquainted with Latin).

The boarding-school occupied a fine old-fashioned mansion. The noble drawing-room, with its numerous windows overlooking the bay, was the scene of my teaching duties.

When they were over, many quiet hours were passed in that pleasant room, studying the medical books which the Doctor supplied from his library.

The severe duties of teaching and study were occasionally varied by larger interests, such as hearing a very able (though erroneous) oration on States' Rights, by Calhoun; or the more carnal pleasure of a visit to a banana plantation.

John C. Calhoun's address, given to the enthusiastic meeting which crowded the theatre, was note-worthy. The contrast between the calm, able orator, who appeared entirely unmoved by the rapturous demonstrations of his audience, who responded to every point in his clever but measured oratory, resembled the effect produced in our later day by the able statesman Parnell, who dominated his ardent Irish followers by a similarly contrasted mental constitution. The influence of this able statesman, John C. Calhoun, was largely instrumental in causing the Civil War in America.

The following familiar home letters indicate some of the varieties in the Charleston life:—

Charleston: January 30, 1847.

Now, dear M., for a comfortable Sunday afternoon chat with you, after a long—it seems to me a very long—silence. I've just replenished my body with a comfortable portion of our regular Sunday dinner—viz. ham, fowl, sweet potatoes, and macaroni—of which last I've grown particularly fond, and now, wrapped in my blanket-shawl, I sit with my feet on the fender, over the embers of the parlour fire, and, as the girls are at church and only good Miss B. in the room, I hope for a nice long quiet time. But I must tell you of a great musical treat I've had, really the highest pleasure in that way that I ever remember; no less than two concerts by Herz and Sivori. I never have been so affected by music before; yet the first concert made me sad, homesick, and discontented. I felt as I do after reading a powerful novel of Bulwer's. It was Sivori's violin that produced so strange an effect. Herz was a smooth, brilliant pianoforte player, with considerable superficial talent, nothing more; but Sivori has genius. His playing bewildered me; I did not understand it. It seemed to me like a chaos that might become a world of beauty could I only find the word that should reduce it to order. I went home unhappy and indignant at being obliged to pass life in such a stupid place, amongst such stupid people, where is neither beauty, nor intelligence, nor goodness. The next concert it went better with me. I sat near the platform immediately in front of Sivori, and examined his countenance, which certainly renders his performance clearer. He is very small, his head large for his body, a fine forehead, grand eyes, a stiff, sober manner, and occasional half-suppressed smile that reminded me continually of Ellery Channing. The first piece, "Il Campanello" of Paganini, was a gem; the solemn, subduing *adagio*, with a wild, striving conclusion, and the little clear silver bell coming in continually, like an angel's voice in the conflict of good and bad spirits. Then his prayer from "Moïse," performed on one string, was the most devout music I ever listened to. I felt as if

I were worshipping in an old cathedral at twilight, and I shut my eyes not to destroy the illusion by the expressionless concert-room and faces all round. The duet between Herz and Sivori was grand, both parts were so perfect. I went to the concert with a prejudice against Herz, from knowing his very bad moral character; but his playing is very brilliant, though he is far from being a De Meyer. He has the most self-satisfied expression in his mouth, which, as a gentleman remarked, "seems to be going to eat his ears," it is so large. He was recalled after one of his pieces, and said, smiling, "I will play you a piece which I composed, since I am in Charleston. It is called 'Souvenir de Charleston.'" 'Twas quite a dashing affair; and then he extemporised beautifully on "Lucy Long." I hope you may have the pleasure in Cincinnati of hearing these real artists. Oh for the time when such music may be a daily feast for all, and when the performers shall be as noble in character as they are gifted in talent!

Charleston: February 28, 1847.

MY DEAR MOTHER,—Two letters from you within a twelvemonth seems as extraordinary as it is welcome. I was much gratified by the kind home voices which greeted my birthday. I always think of old family times on that day—the penny for each year which father used laughingly to bestow, and the silver that came after, and then the little children's party, and all the merry old times; but I am quite satisfied that my childhood has gone; I never wish to recall it, happy as it was; I want to be up and doing, not simply enjoying myself; and if I never succeed in accomplishing all my intentions, I mean to have the comfortable assurance that I have tried hard and done my best. Your letter, besides its highly respected religious advice, which I always lay up carefully in a little scented corner of my mind, contains many little interesting domestic items. How I should like to tap at the window some night, while the brilliant solar lamp is illuminating the planets and glorifying the cheerful faces inside, and make you all start as if you saw a ghost, till a most substantial shaking of the hand should convince you to the contrary! We have had a very mild winter on the whole, to my no small delight, for I dreaded the cold exceedingly in this great house, where the wind rushes grievously through every door and window and finds only the ghost of a fire to warm it, and where heavy mists from the ocean chill the very marrow of your bones. I've fortunately had no broken chilblains on my hands this winter, and as I teach in the warmest room in the house, and throw open the shutters to let in all the sunshine, I don't often have to wear my blanket, but get along pretty comfortably. I am teaching at present more than eight hours a day, and you may imagine I get pretty tired by tea-time. Such a press of teaching, however, will not last very long, and I am quite willing that Mrs Du Pré should gain as much as possible by me while I am with her.

About a week ago I received an answer from the old Quaker physician, Dr. Warrington of Philadelphia, to whom I was introduced by Mrs. Willard of Troy some time ago. The letter is quite an original; I must transcribe a little for your benefit:—

"MY DEAR E. BLACKWELL,—Thy letter of November 18 came duly to hand; it has indeed remained unanswered, but not unheeded. I have reflected much on the propositions contained in it; so strong a hold has the communication had on my feelings and sympathies that I feared I might speak imprudently if I should reply impromptu to such noble sentiments. I have myself been so circumstanced in life as to be rendered measurably competent to understand the force of promptings to move in somewhat new and little-tried paths. My immediate response would therefore perhaps have been, 'Go onwards'; and though if in reasonings with flesh and blood in this matter I may appear less ardent in my encouragement, let it be borne in mind that He who puts forth can without fail lead His devoted servants; He can make a way where there appeared to be no way; He can accomplish

His purposes by instruments of His own selection in the bringing about His own ends—'God shall work, and who shall let (hinder or prevent) Him?'

"Now, this principle is recognisable by the pious of all denominations. It is one which has been found operative in very many important enterprises, and it is one which thy own mind seems so firmly to have settled that I scarcely need advert to it now, but to show that my own faith may sometimes be so feeble that I enter into human calculation as to the expediency of certain plans of operation which have suggested themselves to me in the course of my movements about this great city, or when I am reflecting upon the condition of humanity at large. Now, I frankly confess that it is in such a balance that I have from time to time weighed thy interesting concern. I have personally appealed to some of the most intelligent and liberal-minded ladies of my acquaintance how far the services of a well-educated female physician would be appreciated by them. The response uniformly is, 'Mrs. Gove and Mrs. Wright were unfit to teach, nor could any female become acceptable to us, either as a teacher or practitioner of medicine.' This language is stronger than I should be willing to use myself. It is an interesting matter of history, and one which may afford some encouragement to reformers to persevere, when they are assured that their cause has its foundation in truth, justice, and mercy; that Saul, who had been most bitter in his persecution of Christians, joining in the popular outcry against the great Innovator, not only himself became a convert to the new faith, but under the name of Paul, for the balance of his active life, employed his powerful talents in the extension of the very doctrines which in his misguided zeal he had laboured to subvert. I confess, my dear lady, that I with thee see many difficulties in the way to the attainment—firstly, to the acquisition of the kind and amount of education thou art aware is necessary as a *capital stock* with which to begin the enterprise which has been opened to thy mind; secondly, that after years spent in the attempt the popular mind will be found barred against thy mission of love and humanity; but I beg thee to believe with me that if the project be of divine origin and appointment it will sooner or later surely be accomplished. Thus, in the language of Gamaliel on another occasion, 'If this work be of men it will come to nought, but if it be of God ye cannot overthrow it, lest haply ye be found even to fight against God.' In now addressing thee personally I cordially reiterate the invitation. I should be happy to compare notes with thee at any leisure moment which may be afforded me, though I am in the whirl of occupation; and if after our conferences together thou shouldest become as persuaded as I am that woman was designed to be the helpmeet for man, and that in the responsible duties of relieving ills which flesh is heir to it is appropriate that man be the *physician* and woman the *nurse*, it may possibly occur to thee that thy real mission in this world of probation will be to contribute with all the talents which thy Father in Heaven has so bountifully bestowed the exaltation of a portion of thy sex to the holy duties of nursing the sick, and thus succouring the distressed. With sentiments of most respectful consideration. . . ."

This is a portion of the good Doctor's letter, and though our opinions differ considerably I cannot complain of his treating the matter too lightly. He seems to be an honest, simple-minded, enthusiastic old man, and I feel as if I might regard him as a friend in Philadelphia. The letter is copied by his wife in a clear, pretty hand, so I consider her as interested also.

Well, my dear mother, I wish I could tell you something amusing; but though we do a good deal of small laughing, it would hardly be worth while to put our jokes down on paper. Miss Buell and I talk of hiring a beau if we can get one cheap, for really these beautiful moonlight nights a walk on the Battery would be very pleasant, and a visit to the opera that is now in town would be by no means disagreeable; but now we have to sit at our window and admire the moonlight on the waters, and sigh in vain after the vanities of the world, all for want of a beau—alas! poor nuns that we are. Then sometimes the girls get up a little screaming for our benefit. The other night, for instance, the ten o'clock bell had rung. Miss Buell had seen that the lights were out and the girls in bed. We were comfortably sinking into forgetfulness on our pillows, when I fancied I heard some poor dog yelling in some yard. I listened sympathisingly, and found it was a human voice in the distance uttering at short intervals a succession of agonised shrieks. I was horrified and indignant. "Do listen," I cried; "they must be whipping a poor negro; isn't it abominable?" We listened; the shrieks seemed to draw nearer. "Why, Miss Buell, 'tis certainly the girls in the opposite room!" "Oh, no, they are all asleep; 'tis sonny's voice downstairs: they must be washing him." "At this time of night! What an idea! I'm convinced it is the girls." The shrieks increased, and at intervals we distinguished the words: "Oh, Penny, Penny Grimke! Oh, Miss Buell, Miss Blackwell, Mrs. Peters! Oh, Mrs. Peters!" I jumped out of bed, got a light, and hurried into the opposite room; as I opened the door the noise almost stunned me. There were six girls, all screaming at the top of their voices, as pale as their nightgowns, and some of them almost in fits; all the other doors were thrown open, and I was immediately surrounded by a perfect mob of girls in white nightgowns and caps, talking, crying, laughing, in a regular uproar. I threatened to blow out the lamp, to call Mr. Bonnetheau, to beat them all if they wouldn't hush, and at last I got at the origin of the affray. A couple of brushes had fallen on the floor, and one of the girls, affirming that somebody had touched her arm, began to scream; all the others joined in, and I really believe that if I had not gone to them when I did they would have fallen into convulsions, so completely had they given themselves up to terror. These are some of the pleasant diversions of our life, and as I welcome anything that makes me laugh, they are quite acceptable.

When the hot weather arrived I superintended the summer school, which for the health of the pupils was removed to Aiken,

South Carolina, amongst the pine barrens; a spot renowned for its healthiness, and which has since become a famous health resort.

Aiken: July 1846.

Many happy returns, dear M., of your birthday. I send you the old greeting; old, and full of meaning; for life is a blessing, though our low, unworthy view may make us sometimes doubt it. Even if life were full of suffering, and annihilation its end, I should still hail it as a noble gift. But with a firm faith in infinite goodness and immortality, the most wearisome life becomes a source of triumphant thanksgiving. So I wish you again many happy returns of glorious life! And now I must thank you right heartily for a letter that was a real home gift; or, as the "Dial" saith, "a letter that was no letter, but a leaf out of the book of Nature." How do your commentatical studies go on? I am afraid it will be an unsatisfactory sort of business to search for the sun with a parcel of rushlights; if it do not glow forth with unmistakable brilliancy I fear there's very little true solar light to be found. Last Sunday, not caring to pay the Episcopal church a second visit, I told Mrs. Du Pre I would go to a church in the woods, so she need not send the carriage back for me. I had seen a dark wooden building with little steeple, half hidden amongst the trees, that took my fancy. So I dressed and strolled through the sandy wood paths at the rate of a mile an hour, as I hate overheating myself. I reached my church at length, when, lo! it proved to be a deserted schoolhouse, containing two large cool rooms, built of weather-beaten pine, with projecting roof and pleasant elevated porch. Here I took my seat, whilst the village bells were ringing merrily. The schoolhouse was situated in the midst of pretty woods, encircled by a path of white sand which winds through the woods to the village. The sky was brilliantly blue; the rich odour of the pines and the hum of insects had a very soothing effect, and I spent my time so pleasantly that I think I shall be tempted to pay my church in the woods many visits this summer. By-the-by, I find that the schoolhouse, cool and pleasant as it is, has been for some time deserted, because the three denominations of Aiken cannot agree on the choice of a teacher. I have found the summer here very pleasant hitherto. Indeed, I invite you all to come South and get cool; I think I have never suffered so little from heat anywhere.

November.—Let me set your mind at ease with regard to my fastidiousness, love of beauty, professional horrors, and so forth. My mind is fully made up. I have not the slightest hesitation on the subject; the through study of medicine I am quite resolved to go through with. The horrors and disgusts I have no doubt of vanquishing. I have overcome stronger distastes than any that now remain, and feel fully equal to the contest. As to the opinion of people, I don't care one straw *personally*; though I take so much pains, as a matter of policy, to propitiate it, and shall always strive to do so; for I see continually how the highest good is eclipsed by the violent or disagreeable forms which contain it. I think you attribute a foolish sentimental fastidiousness to me that I do not possess. You also speak of my want of bodily sympathy being an objection. If I understand what you mean, I think it would prove of the most valuable assistance possible. I suspect you were thinking of that unlucky dose of lobelia I once gave you when I grew angry because you groaned and groaned, and obstinately refused to drink the warm stuff that would relieve you. I think I have sufficient hardness to be entirely unaffected by great agony in such a way as to impair the clearness of thought necessary for bringing relief, but I am sure the warmest sympathy would prompt me to relieve suffering to the extent of my power; though I do not think any case would keep me awake at night, or that the responsibility would seem too great when I had conscientiously done my best. . . . I want very much to have a little story printed which I have translated from the German. It is very pretty, and pleases the children greatly. I might get a hundred dollars for it. . . . Aiken is almost deserted, but I shall not go down till the 15th, when the Episcopal minister arrives to take charge of the school. To-morrow I shall be left entirely alone, not a soul in the house besides; and only a negro man somewhat given to drink and a negro woman greatly given to scolding in the yard. . . . The autumn winds are howling round the house, blowing the leaves in whirlwinds. Our "Fall" has been very pleasant, though we've had fires for several weeks. The changing trees had a curious effect for a few days. I have four windows in my room, and the hickory trees outside turned a brilliant yellow, filling the room with a beautiful glow. During a very rainy day I several times looked up with joy thinking the sun was breaking forth; but the rain soon changed their beauty, and now our pines and some oaks are the only cheerful things left.

Returning to Charleston, the winter and spring were fully occupied with teaching; the Christmas being cheered by the receipt from home of our "Family Christmas Annual," a collection of articles in prose and verse, specially prepared anonymously by the various members of the family, and decorated by domestic artists. This diversion was continued for many years; and several volumes are still preserved as mementoes of those pleasant times.

Chapter Three

Study in America

1847–1849

IN the summer of 1847, with my carefully hoarded earnings, I resolved to seek an entrance into a medical school. Philadelphia was then considered the chief seat of medical learning in America, so to Philadelphia I went; taking passage in a sailing vessel from Charleston for the sake of economy.

In Philadelphia I boarded in the family of Dr. William Elder. He and his admirable wife soon became warm and steadfast friends. Dr. Elder (author of the life of Dr. Kane, the Arctic voyager) was a remarkable man, of brilliant talent and genial nature. He took a generous interest in my plans, helping by his advice and encouragement through the months of effort and refusals which were now encountered.

Applications were cautiously but persistently made to the four medical colleges of Philadelphia for admission as a regular student. The interviews with their various professors were by turns hopeful and disappointing. Whilst pursuing these inquiries

I commenced my anatomical studies in the private school of Dr. Allen. This gentleman by his thoughtful arrangements enabled me to overcome the natural repulsion to these studies generally felt at the outset. With a tact and delicacy for which I have always felt grateful, he gave me as my first lesson in practical anatomy a demonstration of the human wrist. The beauty of the tendons and exquisite arrangements of this part of the body struck my artistic sense, and appealed to the sentiment of reverence with which this anatomical branch of study was ever afterwards invested in my mind.

During the following months, whilst making applications to the different medical colleges of Philadelphia for admission as a regular student, I enlisted the services of my friends in the search for an Alma Mater. The interviews with the various professors, though disappointing, were often amusing.

EXTRACTS FROM THE JOURNAL OF 1847

May 27.—Called on Dr. Jackson (one of the oldest professors in Philadelphia), a small, bright-faced, grey-haired man, who looked up from his newspaper and saluted me with, "Well, what is it? What do you want?" I told him I wanted to study medicine. He began to laugh, and asked me why. Then I detailed my plans. He became interested; said he would not give me an answer then; that there were great difficulties, but he did not know that they were insurmountable; he would let me know on Monday. I came home with a lighter heart, though I can hardly say I hope. On Monday Dr. Jackson said he had done his best for me, but the professors were all opposed to my entrance. Dr. Horner advised me to try the Filbert Street and Franklin schools. A professor of Jefferson College thought it would be impossible to study there, and advised the New England schools.

June 2.—Felt gloomy as thunder, trudging round to Dr. Darrach. He is the most non-committal man I ever saw. I harangued him, and he sat full five minutes without a word. I asked at last if he could give me any encouragement. "The subject is a novel one, madam, I have nothing to say either for or against it; you have awakened trains of thought upon which my mind is taking action, but I cannot express my opinion to you either one way or another." "Your opinion, I fear, is unfavourable." "I did not say so. I beg you, madam, distinctly to understand that I express no opinion one way or another; the way in which my mind acts in this matter I do not feel at liberty to unfold." "Shall I call on the other professors of your college?" "I cannot take the responsibility of advising you to pursue such a course." "Can you not grant me admittance to your lectures, as you do not feel unfavourable to my scheme?" "I have said no such thing; whether favourable or unfavourable, I have not expressed any opinion; and I beg leave to state clearly that the operation of my mind in regard to this matter I do not feel at liberty to unfold." I got up in despair, leaving his mind to take action on the subject at his leisure.

Dr. Warrington told me that he had seen his friend Dr. Ashmead, who had told him that Paris was such a horrible place that I must give up my wish for a medical education—indeed, his communication would be so unfavourable that he would rather not meet me in person. I told the Doctor that if the path of duty led me to hell I would go there; and I did not think that by being with devils I should become a devil myself—at which the good Doctor stared.

Nevertheless, I shrink extremely from the idea of giving up the attempt in America and going to France, although the suggestion is often urged on me.

The fear of successful rivalry which at that time often existed in the medical mind was expressed by the dean of one of the smaller schools, who frankly replied to the application, "You cannot expect us to furnish you with a stick to break our heads with"; so revolutionary seemed the attempt of a woman to leave a subordinate position and seek to obtain a complete medical education. A similarly mistaken notion of the rapid practical success which would attend a lady doctor was shown later by one of the professors of my medical college, who was desirous of entering into partnership with me on condition of sharing profits over 5,000 dollars on my first year's practice.

During these fruitless efforts my kindly Quaker adviser, whose private lectures I attended, said to me: "Elizabeth, it is of no use trying. Thee cannot gain admission to these schools. Thee must go to Paris and don masculine attire to gain the necessary knowledge." Curiously enough, this suggestion of disguise made by good Dr. Warrington was also given me by Doctor Pankhurst, the Professor of Surgery in the largest college in Philadelphia. He thoroughly approved of a woman's gaining complete medical knowledge; told me that although my public entrance into the classes was out of the question, yet if I would assume masculine attire and enter the college he could entirely rely on two or three of his students to whom he should communicate my disguise, who would watch the class and give me timely notice to withdraw should my disguise be suspected.

But neither the advice to go to Paris nor the suggestion of disguise tempted me for a moment. It was to my mind a moral crusade on which I had entered, a course of justice and common sense, and it must be pursued in the light of day, and with public sanction, in order to accomplish its end.

The following letter to Mrs. Willard of Troy, the well-known educationalist, describes the difficulties through which the young student had to walk warily:—

Philadelphia: May 24.

I cannot refrain from expressing my obligations to you for directing me to the excellent Dr. Warrington. He has allowed me to visit his patients, attend his lectures, and make use of his library, and has spoken to more than one medical friend concerning my wishes; but with deep regret I am obliged to say that all the information hitherto obtained serves to show me the impossibility of accomplishing my purpose in America. I find myself rigidly excluded from the regular college routine, and there is no thorough course of lectures that can supply its place. The general sentiment of the physicians is strongly opposed to a woman's intruding herself into the profession; consequently it would be perhaps impossible to obtain private instruction, but if that were possible, the enormous expense would render it impracticable, and where the feelings of the profession are strongly enlisted against such a scheme, the museums, libraries, hospitals, and all similar aids would be closed against me. In view of these and numerous other difficulties Dr. Warrington is discouraged, and joins with his medical brethren in advising me to give up the scheme. But a strong idea, long cherished till it has taken deep root in the soul and become an all-absorbing duty, cannot thus be laid aside. I must accomplish my end. I consider it the noblest and most useful path that I can tread, and if one country rejects me I will go to another.

Through Dr. Warrington and other sources I am informed that my plan can be carried out in Paris, though the free Government lectures, delivered by the faculty, are confined to men, and a diploma is strictly denied to a woman, even when (as in one instance, as it is said) she has gone through the course in male attire; yet every year thorough courses of lectures are delivered by able physicians on every branch of medical knowledge, to which I should be admitted without hesitation and treated with becoming respect. The true place for study, then, seems open to me; but here, again, some friendly physicians raise stronger objections than ever. "You, a young unmarried lady," they say, "go to Paris, that city of fearful immorality, where every feeling will be outraged and insult attend you at every step; where vice is the natural atmosphere, and no young man can breathe it without being contaminated! Impossible, you are lost if you go!"

Now, dear madam, I appeal to you, who have had the opportunity of studying the French in their native land, is not this a false view, a greatly exaggerated fear? Is it not perfectly true everywhere that a woman who respects herself will be respected by others; that where the life is directed by a strong, pure motive to a noble object, in a quiet, dignified, but determined manner, the better feelings of mankind are enlisted, and the woman excites esteem and respectful sympathy? To my mind this is perfectly clear, and I trust that your more experienced judgment will confirm my opinion. Probably, then, if all the information which I am still collecting agree with what I have already received, I may sail for France in the course of the summer, that I may familiarise myself with a rapid French delivery before the commencement of the winter lectures.

I have tried to look every difficulty steadily in the face. I find none which seem to me unconquerable, and with the blessing of Providence I trust to accomplish my design.

After a short, refreshing trip with my family to the seaside, the search was again renewed in Philadelphia. But applications made for admission to the medical schools both of Philadelphia and of New York were met with similarly unsuccessful results.

I therefore obtained a complete list of all the smaller schools of the Northern States, "country schools," as they were called. I examined their prospectuses, and quite at a venture sent in applications for admission to twelve of the most promising institutions, where full courses of instruction were given under able professors. The result was awaited with much anxiety, as the time for the commencement of the winter sessions was rapidly approaching. No answer came for some time. At last, to my immense relief (though not surprise, for failure never seemed possible), I received the following letter from the medical department of a small university town in the western part of the State of New York:—

Geneva: October 20, 1847.

To Elizabeth Blackwell, Philadelphia.

I am instructed by the faculty of the medical department of Geneva University to acknowledge receipt of yours of 3rd inst. A quorum of the faculty assembled last evening for the first time during the session, and it was thought important to submit your proposal to the class (of students), who have had a meeting this day, and acted entirely on their own behalf, without any interference on the part of the faculty. I send you the result of their deliberations, and need only add that there are no fears but that you can, by judicious management, not only "disarm criticism," but elevate yourself without detracting in the least from the dignity of the profession.

Wishing you success in your undertaking, which some may deem bold in the present state of society, I subscribe myself,

Yours respectfully,

CHARLES A. LEE,

Dean of the Faculty.

15 Geneva Hotel

This letter enclosed the following unique and manly letter, which I had afterwards copied on parchment, and esteem one of my most valued possessions:—

At a meeting of the entire medical class of Geneva Medical College, held this day, October 20, 1847, the following resolutions were unanimously adopted:—

1. *Resolved*—That one of the radical principles of a Republican Government is the universal education of both sexes; that to every branch of scientific education the door should be open equally to all; that the application of Elizabeth Blackwell to become a member of our class meets our entire approbation; and in extending our unanimous invitation we pledge ourselves that no conduct of ours shall cause her to regret her attendance at this institution.
2. *Resolved*—That a copy of these proceedings be signed by the chairman and transmitted to Elizabeth Blackwell.

T. J. STRATTON, *Chairman*

With an immense sigh of relief and aspiration of profound gratitude to Providence I instantly accepted the invitation, and prepared for the journey to Western New York State.

Leaving Philadelphia on November 4, I hastened through New York, travelled all night, and reached the little town of Geneva at 11 P.M. on November 6.

The next day, after a refreshing sleep, I sallied forth for an interview with the dean of the college, enjoying the view of the beautiful lake on which Geneva is situated, notwithstanding the cold, drizzling, windy day. After an interview with the authorities of the college I was duly inscribed on the list as student No. 130, in the medical department of the Geneva University.

I at once established myself in a comfortable boarding-house, in the same street as my college and three minutes' walk from it—a beautiful walk along the high bank overlooking the lake. I hung my room with dear mementoes of absent friends, and soon with hope and zeal and thankful feelings of rest I settled down to study.

Naturally, some little time was required to adjust the relations of the new student to her unusual surroundings. My first experiences are thus given in a letter to a sister:—

Geneva: November 9, 1847.

I've just finished copying the notes of my last lecture. Business is over for to-day; I throw a fresh stick into my "air-tight," and now for refreshment by a talk with my own dear sister. Your letter containing E.'s was the first to welcome me in my new residence; right welcome, I assure you, it was, for I was gloomy—very. It was on Monday evening your letter came—my first work-day in Geneva. It had rained incessantly; I was in an upper room of a large boarding-house without a soul to speak to. I had attended five lectures, but nevertheless I did not know whether I could do what I ought to, for the Professor of Anatomy was absent, and had been spoken of as a queer man. The demonstrator hesitated as to my dissecting; I had no books, and didn't know where to get any; and my head was bewildered with running about the great college building—never going out of the same door I went in at.

This evening, however, I have finished my second day's lectures; the weather is still gloomy, but I feel sunshiny and happy, strongly encouraged, with a grand future before me, and all owing to a fat little fairy in the shape of the Professor of Anatomy! This morning, on repairing to the college, I was introduced to Dr. Webster, the Professor of Anatomy, a little plump man, blunt in manner and very voluble. He shook me warmly by the hand, said my plan was capital; he had some fun too about a lady pupil, for he never lost a joke; the class had acted manfully; their resolutions were as good as a political meeting, &c.

He asked me what branches I had studied. I told him all but surgery. "Well," said Dr. Lee, "do you mean to practise surgery?" "Why, of course she does," broke in Dr. Webster. "Think of the cases of femoral hernia; only think what a well-educated woman would do in a city like New York. Why, my dear sir, she'd have her hands full in no time; her success would be immense. Yes, yes, you'll go through the course, and get your diploma with great *éclat* too; we'll give you the opportunities. You'll make a stir, I can tell you."

I handed him a note of introduction from Dr. Warrington, and then he told me to wait in the ante-room while he read it to the medical class, who were assembled in the amphitheatre for his lecture, which was to be preparatory to one of the most delicate operations in surgery, and I suppose he wanted to remind them of their promise of good behaviour. I could hear him reading it. When his age and experience were spoken of there was a shout of laughter, for he can't be more than forty-five and not much of dignity about him; but at the conclusion there was a round of applause, after which I quietly entered, and certainly have no reason to complain of medical students, for though they eye me curiously, it is also in a very friendly manner. After the lecture was over, the demonstrator, who now shows the utmost friendliness, explained to me at the Doctor's request a very important subject which I had lost. It was admirably done, illustrated on the subject, and if to-day's lessons were a fair specimen, I certainly shall have no cause to complain of my anatomical instructors. The plan pursued here is admirable, and New York and Philadelphia may learn more than one lesson from Geneva. Dr. Webster came to me laughing after the first lecture, saying: "You attract too much attention, Miss Blackwell; there was a very large number of strangers present this afternoon—I shall guard against this in future." "Yes," said Dr. Lee; "we were saying to-day that this step might prove quite a good advertisement for the college; if there were no other advantage to be gained, it will attract so much notice. I shall bring the matter into the medical journals; why, I'll venture to say in ten years' time one-third the classes in our colleges will consist of women. After the precedent you will have established, people's eyes will be opened."

Now, all this kind feeling encourages me greatly, and I need it; for though my purpose has never wavered, a flat, heavy feeling was growing upon me from constant disappointment. I was fast losing that spring of hope that is so pleasant; consequently praise cannot make me vain, and the notice I attract is a matter of perfect indifference. I sit quietly in this large assemblage of young men, and they might be women or mummies for aught I care. I sometimes think I'm too much disciplined, but it is certainly necessary for the position I occupy. I believe the professors don't exactly know in what species of the human family to place me, and the students are a little bewildered. The other people at first regarded me with suspicion, but I am so quiet and gentle that suspicion turns to astonishment, and even the little boys in the street stand still and stare as I pass. 'Tis droll; sometimes I laugh, sometimes I feel a little sad, but in Geneva the nine days' wonder soon will cease, and I cannot but congratulate myself on having found at last the right place for my beginning.

I had not the slightest idea of the commotion created by my appearance as a medical student in the little town. Very slowly I perceived that a doctor's wife at the table avoided any communication with me, and that as I walked backwards and forwards to college the ladies stopped to stare at me, as at a curious animal. I afterwards found that I had so shocked Geneva propriety that the theory was fully established either that I was a bad woman, whose designs would gradually become evident, or that, being insane, an outbreak of insanity would soon be apparent. Feeling the unfriendliness of the people, though quite unaware of all this gossip, I never walked abroad, but hastening daily to my college as to a sure refuge, I knew when I shut the great doors behind me that I shut out all unkindly criticism, and I soon felt perfectly at home amongst my fellow-students.

The following extracts from my journal of those days show how any early difficulties were successfully overcome:—

November 9.—My first happy day; I feel really encouraged. The little fat Professor of Anatomy is a capital fellow; certainly I shall love fat men more than lean ones henceforth. He gave just the go-ahead directing impulse needful; he will afford me every advantage, and says I shall graduate with *éclat*. Then, too, I am glad that they like the notoriety of the thing, and think it a good "spec."

November 10.—Attended the demonstrator's evening lecture—very clear—how superior to books! Oh, this is the way to learn! The class behaves very well; and people seem all to grow kind.

November 11.—Anatomy very interesting to-day; two admirable demonstrations. Dr. Webster, full of enthusiasm, told us of Godman, who was converted to phrenology by reading a work against it, in order to cut it up.

November 15.—To-day, a second operation at which I was not allowed to be present. This annoys me. I was quite saddened and discouraged by Dr. Webster requesting me to be absent from some of his demonstrations. I don't believe it is his wish. I wrote to him hoping to change things.

November 17.—Dr. Webster seemed much pleased with my note, and quite cheered me by his wish to read it to the class to-morrow, saying if they were all actuated by such sentiments the medical class at Geneva would be a very noble one. He could hardly guess how much I needed a little praise. I have no fear of the kind students.

November 20.—In the amphitheatre yesterday a little folded paper dropped on my arms as I was making notes; it looked very much as if there were writing in it, but I shook it off and went on quietly with my notes. Some after-demonstration of a similar kind produced a hiss from the opposite side of the room. I felt also a very light touch on my head, but I guess my quiet manner will soon stop any nonsense.

November 22.—A trying day, and I feel almost worn out, though it was encouraging too, and in some measure a triumph; but 'tis a terrible ordeal! That dissection was just as much as I could bear. Some of the students blushed, some were hysterical, not one could keep in a smile, and some who I am sure would not hurt my feelings for the world if it depended on them, held down their faces and shook. My delicacy was certainly shocked, and yet the exhibition was in some sense ludicrous. I had to pinch my hand till the blood nearly came, and call on Christ to help me from smiling, for that would have ruined everything; but I sat in grave indifference, though the effort made my heart palpitate most painfully. Dr. Webster, who had perhaps the most trying position, behaved admirably.

November 24.—To-day the Doctor read my note to the class. In this note I told him that I was there as a student with an earnest purpose, and as a student simply I should be regarded; that the study of anatomy was a most serious one, exciting profound reverence, and the suggestion to absent myself from any lectures seemed to me a grave mistake. I did not wish to do so, but would yield to any wish of the class without hesitation, if it *was* their desire. I stayed in the ante-room whilst the note was being read. I listened joyfully to the very hearty approbation with which it was received by the class, and then entered the amphitheatre and quietly resumed my place. The Doctor told me he felt quite relieved.

No further difficulty ever afterwards occurred.

December 4.—Dr. Webster sent for me to examine a case of a poor woman at his rooms. 'Twas a horrible exposure; indecent for any poor woman to be subjected to such a torture; she seemed to feel it, poor and ignorant as she was. I felt more than ever the necessity of my mission. But I went home out of spirits, I hardly know why. I felt alone. I must work by myself all life long.

Christmas Day.—Bright and gay with sleighs. The lake looks most beautiful, the mist rising from it in arches, the sky a brilliant blue, and the ground covered with snow. I received my Christmas Annual with great joy; and having purchased 25 cents' worth of almonds and raisins, I had quite a cosy time reading it.

Sunday, January 16.—A most beautiful day; it did me good. The text impressed itself on me—"Thou wilt keep him in perfect peace whose mind is stayed on Thee." I felt happy and blessed. Ah! if the Almighty would always shine on me, how strong I should be! "The Lord God is a sun and shield; the Lord will give grace and glory; no good thing will He withhold from them that walk uprightly."

The behaviour of the medical class during the two years that I was with them was admirable. It was that of true Christian gentlemen. I learned later that some of them had been inclined to think my application for admission a hoax, perpetrated at their expense by a rival college. But when the *bona-fide* student actually appeared they gave her a manly welcome, and fulfilled to the letter the promise contained in their invitation.

My place in the various lecture-rooms was always kept for me, and I was never in any way molested. Walking down the crowded amphitheatre after the class was seated, no notice was taken of me. Whilst the class waited in one of the large lecture-rooms for the Professor of Practice, groups of the wilder students gathered at the windows, which overlooked the grounds of a large normal school for young ladies. The pupils of this institution knew the hour of this lecture, and gathered at their windows for a little fun. Here, peeping from behind the blinds, they responded to the jests and hurrahs of the students. "See the one in pink!" "No, look at the one with a blue tie; she has a note," &.—fun suddenly hushed by the entrance of the Professor. Meanwhile I had quietly looked over my notes in the seat always reserved for me, entirely undisturbed by the frolic going on at the windows.

My studies in anatomy were most thoughtfully arranged by Dr. Le Ford, who selected four of the steadier students to work with me in the private room of the surgical professor, adjoining the amphitheatre. There we worked evening after evening in the most friendly way, and I gained curious glimpses into the escapades of student life. Being several years older than my companions, they treated me like an elder sister, and talked freely together, feeling my friendly sympathy.

Under the intelligent instruction of the demonstrator anatomy became a most fascinating study. The wonderful arrangements of the human body excited an interest and admiration which simply obliterated the more superficial feelings of repugnance; and I passed hour after hour at night alone in the college, tracing out the ramification of parts, until, suddenly struck by the intense stillness around, I found that it was nearly midnight, and the rest of the little town asleep.

I was equally amazed and shocked some years later, after dining with Mr. Walsh, the American Consul in Paris, to learn that he had remarked that he could not look at my long slender fingers without thinking of the anatomical work in which they had been engaged.

As the term drew to its end there was regret at parting from friends I had made, and also anxiety from the uncertainties that still attended my future course. These feelings are expressed in my journal:—

January 21.—I felt sad when the lectures actually closed. I received a curious friendly letter from one of the students, requesting the honour of an occasional correspondence. It cheered me, funny as it was. Another student told me he had a daguerreotype-room, and asked me to sit for my likeness to-morrow; but I told him it had annoyed me so much to see my name in the papers that I certainly could not give my face too.[1] He said he had thought of graduating in August, but now he was glad he had not, as I intended returning to Geneva—too funny!

January 24.—Went to Dr. Hadley for my certificate; and attended the examinations. I suppose they were as thorough as most; but they were certainly not much of a test. Most of the students answered very well, but some very badly.

Miss Waller gave me an oyster supper and we had a very pleasant time. Mrs. Wilson convulsed us by an account of how she was actually struck down by the sudden braying of a jackass, which she heard for the first time during a visit to the North, she never having heard the bray before.

---

1. I was then very shy, and much annoyed by such public notices as the following:—

"A very notable event of the year 1848 was the appearance at the medical lectures of a young woman student named Blackwell. She is a pretty little specimen of the feminine gender, said the Boston *Medical Journal*, reporting her age at twenty-six. She comes into the class with great composure, takes off her bonnet and puts it under the seat, exposing a fine phrenology. The effect on the class has been good, and great decorum is observed while she is present. The sprightly Baltimore *Sun* remarked that she should confine her practice, when admitted, to diseases of the heart."—*Springfield Republican*.

January 25.—Attended Commencement (or ceremony of graduation), which after all was not so very formidable. When I went to wish Dr. Hadley good-bye I found the whole faculty assembled, and very merry at breaking up. They talked over my affairs, but gave me no important advice. To my great disappointment no letters of introduction were prepared for me, but only a promise given that they should be sent on at once. I was very sad at parting from the Wallers; but had a pleasant chat with the students whom I found in the railroad cars.

Passing through New York, where I dined with my kind preceptor, Dr. S. H. Dickson, and his wife, then living in the town, I returned to Philadelphia to try and arrange for summer study. Whilst seeking medical opportunities I again stayed in Dr. Elder's family, and endeavoured to increase my slender finances by disposing of some stories I had written, and by obtaining music pupils.

Knowing very little of practical medicine, I finally decided to spend the summer, if possible, studying in the hospital wards of the great Blockley Almshouse of Philadelphia. This enormous institution promised a fine field of observation. I obtained a letter of introduction to Mr. Gilpin, one of the directors of the almshouse.

He received me most kindly, but informed me that the institution was so dominated by party feeling that if he, as a Whig, should bring forward my application for admission, it would be inevitably opposed by the other two parties—viz. the Democrats and the Native Americans. He said that my only chance of admission lay in securing the support of each of those parties, without referring in any way to the other rival parties. I accordingly undertook my sole act of "lobbying." I interviewed each political leader with favourable results, and then sent in my petition to the first Board meeting—when, lo! a unique scene took place; all were prepared to fight in my behalf, but there was no one to fight! I was unanimously admitted to reside in the hospital. This unanimity, I was afterwards assured, was quite without precedent in the records of the institution.

On entering the Blockley Almshouse, a large room on the third floor had been appropriated to my use. It was in the women's syphilitic department, the most unruly part of the institution. It was thought that my residence there might act as a check on the very disorderly inmates. My presence was a mystery to these poor creatures. I used to hear stealthy steps approach and pause at my door, evidently curious to know what I was about. So I placed my table with the books and papers on which I was engaged directly in a line with the keyhole; and there I worked in view of any who chose to investigate the proceedings of the mysterious stranger. The following home letter gives a glimpse of the Blockley life:—

August.

DEAR MOTHER,—Do not fear for me. I go on smoothly and healthily at Blockley; there is really nothing pestilential amongst the diseases, and I live simply, do my duty, trust in God, and mock at the devil! The matron is the only lady in the establishment (present company excepted), and I frequently step in to see her. She wears a nice white cap, has smooth grey hair, and soft dove's eyes like yours, and I sometimes look at her and think of you till her loud voice breaks forth in fierce scolding, and then I think of Mrs. Beelzebub. She sits in an immense room, in the centre of the almshouse proper, and ensconced in her armchair, with feet propped on a velvet footstool, she dispenses orders from morning to night, gives out clothing, raves at the paupers, and dooms the refractory ones to a shower-bath. She is a Quaker—very pious, I believe—attends yearly meeting regularly, and has an Episcopal minister for her only son; she is one of the "strong-minded women," and manages matters to the entire satisfaction of the committee. I like to talk with her occasionally, for she is shrewd and has seen much of life through dark spectacles.

What a contrast she is to our head physician! When I first saw Dr. Benedict I thought him the very loveliest man the Almighty ever created, and I still preserve my opinion; the tears come into his eyes as he bends down to soothe some dying woman, and his voice is as gentle, his touch as kind to each patient as if she were his sister. Then he is as truthful, energetic, and spirited as he is kind, so, of course, we are very good friends, though we don't see much of each other.

I often send a thought to Cincinnati as I roam through the wards and imagine our contrasted employments; all letters unite in calling you the best, the most cheerful, most indefatigable mother that ever did exist. "All her daughters praise her, and her sons call her blessed." How I wish you could pay me another visit this summer! Well, dear mother, Heaven bless you—write to me sometime.

Your loving physician, E.

At that time, and for many years after, the subject which those wards where I lived represented was an unknown problem to me. I was strangely ignorant of the extent and meaning of that phase of our human society which represents the selfish relations of men and women. This semi-blindness, however, proved a real safeguard to me through the many unusual experiences of my subsequent life. It was not until 1869, when attending the Social Science Congress in Bristol, that my mind at last fully comprehended the hideousness of modern fornication.

But my residence at Blockley prepared my mind to some extent for later revelations, as is shown by entries in my journal:—

June 22.—I had a long talk with Nurse Welch, on the patients in her departments, which impressed me deeply. Most of the women are unmarried, a large proportion having lived at service and been seduced by their masters, though, on the whole, about as many seducers are unmarried as married; I found no instance of a married woman living with her husband entering.

This morning one young woman tried to escape from Blockley by tying sheets together and fastening them outside the window bars, but they giving way, she fell down from the third storey, and was picked up suffering from concussion of the brain and other injuries. All this is horrible! Women must really open their eyes to it. I am convinced that *they* must regulate this matter. But how?

August 17.—Drank tea with the matron, and had a very pleasant time. She excites me, and I influence her. She actually apologised to me for her rough and tyrannical treatment of one of the women.

August 19—A beautiful thought came to me this lovely morning. Emerson says, "Our faith comes to us in moments, our vice is habitual." I never till now could explain this to my satisfaction. It is that the atmosphere of our society, of our daily surroundings, is false; it attracts the demons, they encompass us continually, for we live in their home. The angels have to strive to come to us. But when by a holy inspiration, or an effort of man's nobler nature, he rises to a purer sphere, then the angels throng lovingly round him: he breathes the Divine life. But the moment this effort is relaxed, he, not living in a heavenly atmosphere, naturally and inevitably sinks again into hell, because his present home is there—for he cannot separate himself from the race. Not till the *race* is redeemed will our habitual state be heavenly, and the true spontaneous Divine life be possible. This is the philosophy of effort. The solidarity of our race asserts the impossibility of present permanent Divine life. Bless God for our deep momentary experiences—our prophetic assurances! This sweet morning refreshes me inexpressibly. The wind that lifts my hair seems filled with angel hands that soothe the soul to peace; that little warbling bird fills me with holy joy; a glory seems to rest everywhere, a tide from the Divine Nature.

During my residence at Blockley, the medical head of the hospital, Dr. Benedict, was most kind, and gave me every facility in his power. I had free entry to all the women's wards, and was soon on good terms with the nurses. But the young resident physicians, unlike their chief, were not friendly. When I walked into the wards they walked out. They ceased to write the diagnosis and treatment of patients on the card at the head of each bed, which had hitherto been the custom, thus throwing me entirely on my own resources for clinical study.

During the summer of 1848 the famine fever was raging in Ireland. Multitudes of emigrants were attacked with fever whilst crossing the ocean, and so many were brought to Blockley that it was difficult to provide accommodation for them, many being laid on beds on the floor. But this terrible epidemic furnished an impressive object-lesson, and I chose this form of typhus as the subject of my graduation thesis, studying in the midst of the poor dying sufferers who crowded the hospital wards. I read my thesis to Dr. Elder, and was greatly encouraged by his hearty approbation.

Trying as my painful residence at Blockley had been both to body and inind, I was conscious of the great gain in medical knowledge and worldly experience which it had afforded. The following journal entry expresses the mixed feelings with which that strange residence was left:—

September 22.—My last evening at Blockley. Here I sit writing by my first fire. How glad I am, to-morrow, to-morrow, I go home to my friends! And yet as I watched the beautiful sunset from my great windows, as little Mary Ann pays her willing attendance, and all seems so friendly; as I walked to Dr. Benedict's with my thesis, and felt the entrancing day and the lovely country, I *almost* regretted that I was going to leave. Heaven guide me! May good spirits ever surround me!

At the end of the summer I gladly returned to the healthy and hopeful college life at Geneva. Passing through New York, where I saw Dr. Dickson and his family and heard Henry Ward Beecher preach, I reached my winter's home on October 3, reported myself at college, met everywhere a kind welcome, and settled down for winter work. The clever demonstrator again afforded me his valuable aid in anatomy, and the friendliness of the class continued. Sometimes, whilst sitting by the Doctor during some delicate demonstration of the brain, the students who were crowding round, standing on chairs, leaning on one another's shoulders, kept most respectfully from me, drawing back instantly when by accident they touched my head or shoulder.[2]

October 26.—The class held a meeting to-day to request a holiday on election day; and a political division was called for by the assembled students. I went over to the "Free Soil" side, and was received with repeated cheering. I asked Dr. Le Ford, reproachfully, if he was going to vote for the slave-holder, Taylor; whereupon he gave me his

2. See Appendix I.

reasons for political action, and grew quite eloquent in his self-defence.

November 12.—Howy made his appearance to-day, just as I settled down to perpetrate an essay for the family Christmas Annual. How good it is to see a brother! He looked very well, and we had a merry time together. I stayed away from afternoon lectures to be with him. He is a capital companion and greatly improved. I did more laughing than I've done for months. His visit did me real good, for I have been so lonely. Heaven bless the dear boy in his future!

Sunday, 19*th*.—Alone all day in my room, yet anything but lonely. Bright visions of usefulness have been floating round me. I consecrated myself anew to the accomplishment of a great idea. I tried to lecture for an hour to an imaginary audience; striving to prepare for work by seeking expression for my thoughts.

I would I were not so exclusively a doer; speech seems essential to the reformer, but mine is at present a very stammering, childish utterance.

26th.—Went to church. Mr. Hogarth said some true things. He drew our thoughts to the reformers of old, with their sublime trust in the Most High. With a strange feeling of pleasure I claimed kindred with Asa, King of Judah, who broke the idols of the people and overcame the hosts of the Ethiopians.

November 30.—Our evening lecture broke up in a political Hurrah! for a Whig orator and John Van Buren were both speaking in the town, and the students rushed to attend the political meetings. I again discussed the subject with Dr. Le Ford; he justifying himself enthusiastically for being a Whig. He talked well, but I grew tired of those old expediences.

By this time the genuine character of my medical studies was fully established.

Had I been at leisure to seek social acquaintance, I might have been cordially welcomed. But my time was anxiously and engrossingly occupied with studies and the approaching examinations. I lived in my room and my college, and the outside world made little impression on me.

EXTRACTS FROM THE JOURNAL

December 22.—The deepest snow I have seen for years. It was as much as I could do to walk to college; but all was pleasant, the class seem so very friendly. One set me a chair, another spoke so pleasantly, and I had several little friendly chats. How little they know my sensitiveness to these trifling tokens! The unusual weather, an alarm of fire, Dr. Webster's arrival, were so many points for sociability.

December 31.—The New Year's Eve. Alone, as usual, I spent the day; at night, as I watched the last moments of the year slowly depart, a deep solemnity came over me—a hopeless sorrow for poor humanity. I seemed to hear the heavy resounding bell of time, tolling mournfully the dying year, whilst angels with covered faces, and forms that bent with sorrow, waited to receive the finishing scroll of the world's existence, that the fearful record guarded in darkness and silence might at last be unrolled in the terrible light of eternity!

January 1.—Stayed quietly in my room, whilst the merry sleigh-bells and gay voices rang without.

11*th*.—I called to see the pretty blind girl operated on this morning; she was all alone in the hotel, her friends far away. Poor child! she has no protector, within or without; she asked me who the student was that brought her home, when college would be out, &c.; her simple heart and idle fancy are soon caught. Such are the women I long to surround with my stronger arm. Alas! how almost hopeless does the task seem! But God is omnipotent.

January 19.—Dear M.,—I sit down to try and quiet myself by writing to you for this morning. I, as first on the list of candidates, passed through the usual examinations, presented my certificates, received the testimony of satisfaction from the faculty, whose recommendation will procure me the diploma next Tuesday. Now, though the examinations were not very formidable, still the anxiety and effort were as great as if everything were at stake, and when I came from the room and joined the other candidates who were anxiously awaiting their turn, my face burned, my whole being was excited, but a great load was lifted from my mind. The students received me with applause—they all seem to like me, and I believe I shall receive my degree with their united approval; a generous and chivalric feeling having conquered any little feelings of jealousy. I often feel when I am with them how beautiful the relations of man and woman might be under a truer development of character, in nobler circumstances. I do not know the moral character of any one of our students, for I have no genius for hunting up the darker parts of a person's soul; but I know that Geneva is a very immoral place, the lower classes of women being often worthless, the higher ones fastidious and exclusive, so that there is no healthy blending of the sexes. But notwithstanding the bad associations in which they may have been brought up, I have never had any difficulty in giving the right tone to our intercourse. I am more convinced than ever that Fourier is right in placing this matter in the hands of women, and my hope rises when I find that the inner heart of the human being may still remain pure, notwithstanding some corruption of the outer coverings. I don't know if I've ever told you how deep this matter of licentiousness has gradually sunk into my soul, and that the determination to wage a war of extermination with it strengthens continually, and the hope of gaining power and experience to do it worthily is one of my strongest supports in action. So help me God, I will not be blind, indifferent, or stupid in relation to this matter, as are most women. I feel specially called to act in this reform when I have gained wisdom for the task; the world can never be redeemed till this central relation of life is placed on a truer footing.

But I meant to talk to you about the cholera. Our physicians confessedly cannot cure it. The Professor who lectured upon it yesterday commenced: "Gentlemen, I wish I could tell you how to cure the cholera, but under all modes of treatment the mortality seems to be the same; however, I will tell you something of the disease, and what I would do if called to a case."

The cordial relations with Professor and students continued. Throughout the examination time the most friendly interest was felt in my success by my fellow-students. One of my brothers came on to Geneva to attend my graduation. Being personally a stranger to the students, he was much amused by the free indications of friendly comradeship which he overheard. The ceremony of conferring the full and equal diploma of Doctor of Medicine upon a woman excited much interest in the neighbourhood. It was held in the large Presbyterian Church, which, with its ample galleries, was crowded in every part with spectators. The other students walked in procession from the college to the church, but I went up with my brother and took my seat in the side aisle.

EXTRACTS FROM THE JOURNAL OF 1849

January 22.—Our examinations came off successfully. Hurrah, 'tis almost over!

Tuesday, January 23, 1849.—The day, the grand day, is nearly finished; and now whilst visitors are dropping in I must record my first entrance into public life—'twas bright and beautiful and very gratifying. Great curiosity was felt. As I entered and sat in the church I gave one thought to friends, and then thought only of the Holy One. After the degree had been conferred on the others, I was called up alone to the platform. The President, in full academical costume, rose as I came on the stage, and, going through the usual formula of a short Latin address, presented me my diploma. I said: "Sir, I thank you; it shall be the effort of my life, with the help of the Most High, to shed honour on my diploma." The audience applauded, but their presence was little to me. I was filled with a sense of the grandeur of a holy life, with high resolves for the future. As I came down, George Field opened the door of the front row, and I was much touched by the graduates making room for me, and insisting that I should sit with them for the remainder of the exercises. Most gladly I obeyed the friendly invitation, feeling more thoroughly at home in the midst of these true-hearted young men than anywhere else in the town. I heard little of what was said; my whole soul was absorbed in heavenly communion. I felt the angels around me. Dr. Lee gave the valedictory address; he surprised me by the strong and beautiful way in which he alluded to the event. I felt encouraged, strengthened to be greatly good. As I stood at the door the faculty all most kindly wished me good-bye, and Dr. Hale and Bishop De Lancy shook hands and congratulated me. All the ladies collected in the entry, and let me pass between their ranks; and several spoke to me most kindly.

For the next few hours, before I left by train, my room was thronged by visitors. I was glad of the sudden conversion thus shown, but my past experience had given me a useful and permanent lesson at the outset of life as to the very shallow nature of popularity.

The following letter, written by a younger brother who came to be with me on this important occasion, gives some interesting as well as amusing details of the event:—

Geneva: January 23, 1849.

BELOVED RELATIONS.—The important crisis is past, the great occasion over, the object of so much and so justifiable anticipation has been attained, and proud as I always feel of the Blackwells, my familism never seemed to me so reasonable and so perfectly a matter of course as it did this morning, when, having escorted E. into the crowded church and taken my seat beside her, we learned from the music that the graduating class, headed by the dean, trustees, faculty, &c., were marching in solemn conclave into the aisle. I found E. well and in good spirits, as you may suppose. Monday morning E. and I went to the college, where she underwent a second examination, as did also the other members of the graduating class, from the curators of the university, no others but themselves, the class, and the faculty being admitted. From this, as from the former one, our Sis came off with flying colours and the reputation of being altogether the leader of the class. In the afternoon they were successively called upon to read from their theses, and to this I was admitted; but Elizabeth's being in Buffalo to be printed, she could not be called upon. The Professor and students all seem to feel most kindly and warmly friendly. While I sat by the stove on Monday morning at the college whilst the graduating class were undergoing their examination below, the other students, scarcely any of them being acquainted with my personality, conversed freely about matters and things, and of course about Elizabeth. "Well, boys," one would say, "our Elib. feels first-rate this morning. Do you notice how pleased she looks?" "Yes, indeed," replied another, "and I think she well may after the examination she passed yesterday." "So Lizzie will get her diploma after all," said a third. "If any member of the class gets one, *she* is sure of it," said a fourth. Then all agreed that "our Elib." was "a great girl," and in short I found that she was a universal favourite with both professors and students. Nothing could be more cordial than the former are, and several are very gentlemanly and intelligent men indeed, and I formed some pleasant acquaintances among them.

On the morning of the Commencement little Dr. Webster was *in his glory*; he is a warm supporter of Elizabeth and likes a fuss, and nothing could exceed his delight when he found that the whole country round was sending in large numbers of people, and that all the ladies of Geneva were turning out *en masse* to see a lady receive a medical diploma. At ten o'clock A.M. the students met at the college and marched in procession with music to the Literary College, where they were headed by the Bishop of New York, Dr. Hale, the dean, and the curators, the faculty, &c. Dr. Webster was very anxious that E. should march in procession, and sent down two messages to that effect; but E. very properly refused. About half-past ten o'clock Elizabeth and I walked up to the church—she was very nicely dressed in her black brocaded silk gown, *invisibly green* gloves, black silk stockings, &c. As we ascended the college steps, Dr. Webster met Eliz. and again urged the request, whereupon she told him peremptorily that "it wouldn't be ladylike." "Wouldn't it indeed? Why, no, I forgot—I suppose it wouldn't," said the little Doctor, evidently struck for the first time with the idea. So it was arranged that Eliz. and I should sit down at the entrance of the left aisle and join the procession as it came up, and we then walked in and sat down. We found the church, galleries and all, *crowded with ladies*, they only having been as yet admitted; and of course when we came in there was a general stir and murmur, and everybody turned to look at us. By the time the procession came up, all the pews, except those reserved for students, were filled, and the gentlemen had to pour in afterwards and take the aisles, &c. When the procession entered, Mr. Field, a very pleasant, gentlemanly fellow-graduate, offered his arm, and all the class took their seats together in front of the stage. After a short discourse by Dr. Hale, the President, the diplomas were conferred—four being called up at a time—and, ascending the steps to the platform, the President, addressed them in a

Latin formula, taking off his hat, but remaining seated, and so handed them their diplomas, which they received with a bow and retired. Elizabeth was left to the last and called up alone. The President taking off his hat, rose, and addressing her in the same formula, substituting *Domina* for *Domine*, presented her the diploma, whereupon our Sis, who had walked up and stood before him with much dignity, bowed and half turned to retire, but suddenly turning back replied: "Sir, I thank you; by the help of the Most High it shall be the effort of my life to shed honour upon your diploma"; whereupon she bowed and the President bowed, the audience gave manifestations of applause, little Dr. Webster rubbed his hands, the learned curators and faculty nodded grave approbation at each other upon the platform, and our Sis, descending the steps, took her seat with her fellow-physicians in front. Now walks up into the pulpit Professor Lee, with a large manuscript and a solemn air, and commences his address to the graduates. It was on the whole good; he gave it pretty strong to Homœopathists, Hydropathists, Mesmerists, Thompsonians, &c., and gave the ladies of the audience quite a lecture for their encouragement and circulation of quack medicines, informing them that they had better study a little the principles of medicine before attempting to practise what they were so profoundly ignorant about. At the close he alluded to the novel proceeding which they had taken, and the censure or imitation which it would necessarily create. He justified the proceeding, and passed a most gratifying and enthusiastic encomium on the result of the experiment in the case of Eliz. He pronounced her the *leader* of her class; stated that she had passed through a thorough course *in every department*, slighting none; that she had profited to the very utmost by all the advantages of the institution, and by her ladylike and dignified deportment had proved that the strongest intellect and nerve and the most untiring perseverance were compatible with the softest attributes of feminine delicacy and grace, &c., to all which the students manifest by decided attempts at applause their entire concurrence. As the audience passed out the Bishop came up with Dr. Hale, requested an introduction, and spoke very pleasantly, congratulating her on her course, to the great astonishment of the conservatives. As we walked out of the church we found that almost all the ladies had stopped outside, and as we appeared, opened their ranks and let us pass, regarding E. with very friendly countenances. Most of E.'s time was taken up till our departure next day at half-past one o'clock in receiving calls from her few friends.

The admission of a woman for the first time to a complete medical education and full equality in the privileges and the responsibilities of the profession produced a widespread effect in America. The public press very generally recorded the event, and expressed a favourable opinion of it.

Even in Europe some notice of it was taken, and "Punch" showed his cordial appreciation by his amusing but friendly verses.[3]

I knew, however, that a first step only had been taken. Although popular sanction had been gained for the innovation, and a full recognised status secured, yet much more medical experience than I possessed was needed before the serious responsibilities of practice could be justly met. Returning, therefore, to Philadelphia, I endeavoured still to continue my studies. I was politely received by the heads of the profession in Philadelphia as a professional sister, and made the following notes in a journal of that date:—

March 6.—A morning of great gratification; welcomed cordially to the university, and afterwards heard Doctors Jackson, Hodges,

3. See Appendix II.

Gibson, Chapman, and Horner lecture. Drs. Lee and Ford were with me, the former quite in spirits at my reception.

March 10.—Heard Dr. Williamson lecture and received his ticket. Visited the Pennsylvania Hospital, Dr. Levich showing me over it; admired the gallery with its alcoves and the excellent ventilation. I heard Professor Agassiz last night. He has just commenced a course of lectures on the animal world; his manner was simple and earnest, and the principle he laid down will render his course of lectures very interesting if he develop them fully. I am also rubbing up my French, which may be very important to me.

The following letter is characteristic of that period of life:—

February 25.

My Dear Mother.—You sent me a dear, good, welcome letter, and I kiss you heartily for all its affection and sympathy in my eccentric course. I did not miss out, either, any of the pious parts, but I do think, mother mine, that it is a little hard that you will not believe me when I tell you so seriously that my soul is doing first-rate. You urge upon me the importance of religion—why, bless the dear mother, what am I doing else but living religion all the time? Isn't it my meat and my drink to do the good will of God; didn't I use to sit in the lecture-room and send up a whole cannonade of little prayers; and didn't a whole flood of answers come straight down from the throne of grace? And what am I doing now? Do you think I care about medicine? Nay, verily, it's just to kill the devil, whom I hate so heartily—that's the fact, mother; and if that isn't forming Christ in one, the hope of Glory, why, I don't know what is. So pray comfort yourself, and have faith that such a "child of many prayers" will be fixed up all straight at last. . . . I live in a good society, the fellowship of hard-workers, for however little result of my actions may be, I have the strengthening conviction that my aim is right, and that I, too, am working after my little fashion for the redemption of mankind. I agree with you fully in distrusting the "Harbinger," and should certainly banish it from my centre table if I had risen to the dignity of possessing one. I dislike their discussions, and their way of discussing some subjects. I think them calculated to do a great deal of mischief, and am only consoled by the reflection that few people read them. I go in wholesouledly for the Divine marriage institution, and shall always support it by precept, and as soon as I get the chance by example too, and all those who would upset it I consider fools and infidels. I think Associationists too often a very poor set of people, and if they would commence by reforming themselves, and let the Almighty take care of the world, I think they would be much better employed. As to the infidel French philosophy you talk of, it is just twaddle, which I should instantly reject if anybody were to stuff it into me. I am now longing to be at work abroad, where I might spend my time much more profitably—but I do want greatly to see you all again. How long it is since I was at home!—more than five years, I think. I cannot consent to become a stranger to the *Geschwistern*, and W. and E. & E. seem almost unknown. Good-bye, dear mother. I shall see you soon, and then you will be able to read me sermons to your heart's content.—Your M.D.

I felt, however, keenly the need of much wider opportunities for study than were open to women in America. Whilst considering this problem I received an invitation from one of my cousins, then visiting America, to return with him to England, and endeavour to spend some time in European study before engaging in practice in America. This valuable offer was joyfully accepted, and I prepared for a journey to Europe, first of all paying a short farewell visit to my family in Cincinnati.

EXTRACTS FROM THE JOURNAL

April 5.—How kind and good and glad to see me they all were! I walked out with S. and met them all. G. had quite grown out of my knowledge. I am very glad to have spent this fortnight at home. We had general and private talks without end.

April 7.—They all came down to see me off. They stood on the adjoining boat as we sailed away up the river, mother leaning on S., the three sisters on one side, H. and G. on the other, all hearts in sympathy. I could not keep down the tears as I caught the last glimpse of those dear, true ones.

Travelling East, I joined my cousin in Boston, whence we sailed for Liverpool.

EXTRACTS FROM THE JOURNAL

April 18.—Dear Mr. Channing was with me till I left. His medical uncle, Dr. Channing, also came to see me. I never met my old friend more fully; he regretted deeply this flying visit, which disappointed him in the talks he had planned. Beautiful Boston Bay vanished in the distance. America, that land of memories, was left far behind. I took to my berth and lay there in misery five days and nights. How I loathe the ship!

Chapter Four

Study in Europe

1849–1851

ON April 30 we landed at Liverpool, and I began to make acquaintance with the wonderful and unknown Old World, which I had left when a child of eleven. Everything seemed new and striking. The substantial character of Liverpool, the "finished look" of the surrounding country, the extraordinary character of the mining district—all awakened keen interest. My poor cousin being ill with rheumatism, however, we journeyed on at once to his home at Portway Hall, near Dudley. A fortnight was spent in this pleasant home, which, though in the centre of the "Black Country," was surrounded by gardens where the flowers were fresh and sweet, the trees in beautiful leaf, whilst the cuckoo saluted us in the morning and the nightingales at night. I gained a glimpse of the lovely English country, and spent a memorable time in examining the novel surroundings of the great mining district of England. The following letters are descriptive of a young student's impressions on revisiting her native land more than a generation ago.

Portway: May 2, 1849.

Thanks be to Heaven, I am on land once more, and never do I wish again to experience that hideous nightmare—a voyage across the ocean. We had the warmest welcome at my cousin's pleasant home. . . . I went one afternoon to see the casting—that is, when the melted iron, like a river of fire, flows into the moulds which shape it. The Russell Hall Works are close by the town of Dudley. There is a wide extent of smoky country, with many little groups of machinery and brick buildings, each constituting or rather surrounding a pit; many mounds of glowing coal turning into coke; piles of ironstone being burned previous to the smelting; the houses of the managers in various directions, the office at the entrance; and immediately in front the two great blast-furnaces, which burn incessantly day and night, making many thousands of tons a year. Very few workmen were to be seen, but underground a whole army of them were hard at work. The casting was very curious. Twice a day the melted iron is drawn off from the bottom of the great brick towers they call furnaces. Strong men with faces as black and scorched as a coal were busy, armed with iron poles, guiding the sea of fire that rushed out into the moulds that covered a great extent of ground drawing out the white-hot massess of cinders and dirt, and splashing cold water over the front of the furnace to enable them to stand there. We remained at the farther end, but the heat was so great that we had to cover our faces. Suddenly, with a loud noise, the flames burst out from the furnaces, ascending to the very tip, immense volumes of black smoke rolled over our heads, and the rushing noise grew louder and louder. I thought some accident had occurred, and looked out for the safest retreat, when I found it was only the clearing of the furnaces by sending a powerful blast through them, which was always practised after a casting. Within a square of twelve miles one-sixth of the iron used in the world is said to be made. . . . I paid a visit to Dudley Castle, having a great curiosity to see a veritable old castle, a ruined castle; and I explored every corner, looked up the broad chimneys, and peeped out of the stone window frames and loopholes with a feeling of true antiquarian enthusiasm. We sat down on a stone bench at the foot of the keep, which is very old, and on a little hill on the western side of the courtyard; there we tried to revive the scene as it may have looked hundreds of years ago, when armed men were bustling about the court, and visions of fair ladies gleaming from the upper windows and now ruined terraces. The castle crowns a wooded hill, commanding the town and level country for many miles; the remains of a double wall with a moat between still surround the castle. As I stood by those strong walls and looked down on the wide fields below, I began to imagine how grandly an army would approach, and how noble a defence the castle would make, till I longed to revive the ancient conflicts, and almost frightened my companions by my martial demonstrations and visions of grim warriors peeping through the iron-barred windows. But the illusion could not last long; the country is covered with smoke and coal-pits, the wallflower is smiling on the ruins of the old castle, and instead of subterranean dungeons and dark passages the hill is excavated for limestone; and these artificial caverns of enormous extent, with a canal winding through them and echoing to the voices of the workmen, form one of the most curious features of the place, and show how the same energy and power are still at work, though in a very different direction. We drove home through the little town of Dudley, which presented a most curious spectacle, for it was market day, and the workmen from all the country round, having received their wages, were come in with their wives and children to make their weekly purchases. The streets were crammed with people, and our carriage made its way through a living mass that hardly opened to let it through. I examined the people, as I have constantly done since I enterd the country, with great curiosity. I could not see one handsome face in the whole multitude—indeed, the English appear to me a very common-looking people—but neither was I struck by the misery I expected to see. In Liverpool I had peered into all the back alleys and odd corners I could find; I have done the same in Dudley. There is great cleanliness observed everywhere, that compares most favourably with American cities, and the inhabitants of those districts, though miserable, of course, according to a true standard of human life, were neither more numerous nor more wretched than I have been accustomed to see in America. I have very rarely seen a beggar, and in no instance one that has particularly excited my compassion. This district is one of the most thickly peopled in England, and certainly presents an average view of the mining districts, and the poor labourers seem far more comfortable and intelligent than I had supposed. The manufacturing districts, I have no doubt, would present a different spectacle. I have had no opportunity of judging them. I have just learned to my great satisfaction that Mr. Charles Plevins, an old friend of my cousin, is going to London for a few days, and will escort me there and remain during my stay. I can hardly tell what a relief this is, for the idea of going to that great city an entire stranger, and wandering about it utterly alone, was a most desolate, oppressive thought, and entirely destroyed all the pleasure of the anticipation, though I assumed a very independent tone in speaking of my journey when I found it was utterly impossible for cousin to accompany me. He is an old friend of cousin's, though young—only twenty-five—and there is an air of youth and immaturity about all his opinions and actions; but his spirit is so beautiful that you have only to see in order to love it, so pure and gentle, so true and genial. In my opinion he belongs to a class of young Englishmen that I find is large and constantly increasing. Cousin S. is one of them. They are reformers in spirit, but not destroyers; they have no clear immediate plan of reform, and so earnestly maintain the present system until they find a better one; but they are all the time seeking for truth, and longing most earnestly to realise that grand future in which they all believe. Fichte is one of their favourite teachers; Carlyle, Emerson, Channing, all we have known and learned from in the past, they worship now; but they have yet to study Fourier and Swedenborg before they can reach that strong hope and clear insight which will make their working strong, happy, and practically efficient. Now, there is too much of metaphysical abstraction in their thoughts, their religious faith is not a glorious reality, and in the case of our friend Charles, he despises the material world too much, and seeks to subdue the body and purify the spirit by privations which proceed from the noblest motive but a mistaken faith.

I have a curious interest in seeing and hearing him; it revives so completely my earlier life, when I thought as he does now, and strove for the same ends by the same means. My medical effort won his admiration before I arrived, and since I came here he has done me every little service in his power. His family is an old and highly respected one in Birmingham, and when he found I wished to see something of medicine in the city he used his influence to arrange a useful day for me. Accordingly, the day before yesterday I went in with him to Birmingham, having received invitations from several physicians. We spent the day in visiting the various institutions together, and as it was my first introduction to the English medical world, and as I consider it a good omen, I must describe our doings particularly.

Mr. Parker, surgeon to the Queen's Hospital, had some difficulty in believing that it was not an ideal being that was spoken of; but when he found I was really and truly a living woman he sent me an invitation to witness the amputation he was going to perform, and promised to show me all the arrangements of the institution, sending a note of admission to the college and museum. Dr. Evans, a distinguished physician, invited me to the General Hospital, the largest and oldest one, and expressed much sympathy in my undertaking. Dr. McKay, of the Lying-in Hospital, thought that God and Nature had indicated the unfitness of women for such a pursuit as I had chosen, but still said he would be very happy to show the lady all he could. All the students were on the *qui vive* to see the lady surgeon, and as we approached the building I saw them peeping through doors and windows. Mr. Parker, a fat, rosy-faced John Bull, received me very politely, introduced me to some M.D.'s who had come to see the sight, showed me the arrangements of the hospital, which is young and not particularly interesting, and then took me to the operating-room. It was crammed with students, and as fresh ones arrived they would peep about, whisper to their neighbours, and then work their way to a place where they could see me. It was just a repetition of old scenes; a few minutes' curiosity, and then all went on as usual. The students presented the same mixture of faces as our American ones, wore rather better coats, and seemed to be quicker in their movements. I noted nothing peculiar in the operation, which was skilfully performed, without chloroform, which Mr. Parker disliked. Before leaving, he offered me a letter to the famous Roux of Paris.

At the General Hospital, established sixty years, Dr. Heslop received me with the utmost deference, showed me every ward, male and female, pointed out every case of note, let me examine it, and detailed the treatment, particularly one operation for subclavian aneurism, which was so remarkable that they were going to publish the case. Dr. Percy, of Birmingham, a particular friend of S., has promised to meet me in London, and to furnish me with all the necessary introduction to give me an insight into the medical world of the great metropolis. So I look forward now with great hope to a short but delightful visit, and leave for London next Saturday, the 12th, to await my passports, which I shall probably receive with letters on the 16th, and then off again for the land of dancing and wooden shoes. I heard the cuckoo this morning; what a soft human sound it is! Last night the nightingales were singing sweetly in the twilight. Our garden is full of lovely English flowers; the primrose and cowslip, laurustinea, and many others make our garden beautiful, though the weather is a most cold, gloomy nurse to the little darlings.

May 17.—We left Portway yesterday afternoon. I parted from our friends with great regret; we were getting used to one another; a home feeling was growing up there to me, and so it was time to be off. We arrived late in London, so I could only remark the many handsome houses in gardens that marked its environs, the fine and spacious orderly railway station, the wide streets and gay shops. This morning, after seeing Dr. Percy, Cousin S.'s friend, who has promised to give me the necessary introductions to the hospitals to-morrow, we walked about five miles through the city before reaching Mrs. X.'s house in Devonshire Street. During our walk we passed through many handsome squares with monuments and public buildings, not an isolated one, as with us, but row after row of grand pillared edifices, whole streets of palaces, substantial, built of freestone, but all rendered dingy by smoke, which permeates the atmosphere and penetrates everywhere. The most venerable pile of Westminster Abbey is crumbling with age; the cathedral service was being chanted when we entered; the central space was filled with people. The aisles are in the form of a cross, bordered by tall pillars rising lofty and plain to support the long vistas of arches. The spaces are filled up by a wilderness of monuments, a subdued light pouring in, a cool, stony atmosphere filling the cathedral. It is a noble old building, and has impressed me more than anything I've seen. From Westminster Bridge I saw the new Houses of Parliament—an immense pile, the ornaments too delicate for its size. The poor little river was covered with boats, and the bridge with people enjoying the Sunday; but London was much quieter than I supposed it would be. I noticed but one "confectionery store" partly open; the day seemed to be very strictly observed. We walked through Regent Street, and through endless rows of handsome houses constituting the "West End," to Mrs. X.'s. We were shown in by a footman in crimson plush breeches, white stockings, and claret-coloured coat with gold buttons, to the drawing-rooms—the walls lined with figured crimson velvet, and all manner of lounges and tables covered with knick-knackery scattered about. The lady made her appearance in a blue and black satin dress with jet ornaments and a lace head-dress—a handsome brunette, with red cheeks and very black eyes and hair, and altogether too much mannerism to please me. She was evidently criticising me, and holding herself in a noncommittal attitude. I sat still and talked very quietly, thinking to myself that if I were condemned to live there one week I should overturn the lady and smash everything to atoms. Presently a few fashionable morning visitors dropped in to condole with the lady, who had scratched her throat by swallowing a mouthful too hastily, and so was an *invalid*; some messages of inquiry and condolence were delivered by an old, grave footman, so very silly, and answered in so absurd a manner, that I wondered how the man could keep a grave countenance; and yet the lady had wit and spirit which occasionally flashed out. Sir J. H. came in with Dr. H. to see me. I had a little very pleasant talk, and am to meet him on Tuesday. We descended to lunch, ladies sitting down in their bonnets. The dining-room and library had ceilings beautifully painted to imitate the sky with clouds; the whole house was hung with paintings. The lady's manner grew gradually pleasanter; she seemed to like me, admired my hand, and insisted on my drinking a glass of wine—the first I ever took. I told her so, and she was much pleased at her influence. She took us in her barouche through Regent's Park, and then extended her drive to Hyde Park. These parks are very beautiful—miles of grassy lawn, scattered over with groves, gardens, and clumps of trees, with occasional water, and varied with little valleys. They are surrounded by rows of palace houses, sometimes approaching the carriage road, sometimes lost in gardens and shrubbery. I did enjoy to see the people walking about, sitting under the trees, inhaling a little fresh air on the quiet Sunday, for the most perfect order prevailed. Our hostess became quite agreeable, laughed, and chatted merrily about all manner of nothings. It was impossible to converse with her; she must do the talking with a little support, and she gave forth a good deal of shrewd worldly wisdom. She set us down at the Zoological Gardens in Regent's Park, with many regrets that an engagement to a dinner-party in the country prevented her asking me home, and the expression of a strong desire to have a long, full conversation.

Monday, May 1849.—This morning I called on Dr. Carpenter, who has written those admirable works on physiology. He lives near Regent's Park; it was sparkling with dew as I walked through—refreshingly sweet. I found him and his wife exceedingly agreeable. I liked them at once. They questioned me with great interest about my past course. I am to meet some distinguished people at their house to-night, and among them a Miss Gillies, an artist who has watched my steps with the highest pleasure, and who thinks the only true livers are the workers. I received several notes of introduction from Dr. C. He says I must hear Mr. Paget lecture; that he is the most promising surgeon in England. I found an invitation to a pharmaceutical *soirée* awaiting me on my return, with the information that I might see all the distinguished M.D.'s there assembled.

Evening.—I have just returned from Dr. C.'s delightful little party. The ladies were in regular ball costume; some dresses very elegant; dancing to the piano; music, vocal and instrumental. Dr. C. gave us a very beautiful piece of Mendelssohn's on the organ; he and his wife sang together with great feeling. His microscopes, said to be the most beautiful in England, were there. His preparations were exquisite: the lung of a frog most minutely injected, a piece of shark skin which seems covered with innumerable teeth, and piles of other specimens. Miss Gillies is a distinguished artist. I am to visit her and see her relation, Dr. Southwood Smith. Chapman, the well-known publisher, was present, and talked a good deal to me, but seemed a little undecided what tone to take. He has a very handsome, intellectual face. I was introduced to many pleasant people; one had the rare, beautiful face of Cowper's mother. Great interest seemed to be felt in my course.

Before going to Dr. C.'s I went to examine the specimens collected for the pharmaceutical *soirée*. I was surprised to find that the *papier-mâché* models have been hitherto unknown in England, and that the people were regarding with the utmost rapture specimens which are in common use in all American colleges. Sir J. H. drove us to the Consumption Hospital and the Chelsea Botanical Gardens—a most kind-hearted, simple-mannered old gentleman. . . .

Dr. Percy secured me a great treat. I visited the Hunterian Museum in company with Mr. Owen, who lectures at the institution. It is said to be the finest collection of comparative and morbid anatomy in the world. Mr. Owen is a man of genius, and the hour passed away like a minute while listening to his eloquent descriptions of the fossil remains and the laws which related them to living animals, to man, and to the globe. He invited me to come any morning between ten and twelve, but unfortunately my time is too crowded. The obstetric collection is very fine; if I return through London I shall certainly try to spend a week or two in examining it.

We next took the railroad and went to Greenwich, choosing the third-class open cars that I might see the country, which is laid out in market gardens richly cultivated, all round London, though the city, stretching out through Deptford to Greenwich, makes one uninterrupted town in that direction. Greenwich Hospital for Sailors has impressed me more than any other institution with the power and wealth of the nation. It is a series of great palaces, connected by colonnades with double rows of pillars ranged round a large green open to the river, with the park and observatory in the background. The old sailors were hobbling about in comfortable dresses, with enormous rations of bread and meat; for we reached it just at dinner-time, and they were allowed to take their meals and eat in their cabins. There are long walks where they smoke, and they rove about in the freest style. Their chapel is a very beautiful hall, though I fear the rich painting and mosaic is lost on the rough tars. The Painted Hall is immediately opposite; the vaulted ceiling is covered with figures which are larger than life, even from below; the walls are entirely covered with large paintings, richly framed, of naval engagements and naval heroes, and many relics of the great commanders are preserved in cases. The park is always open to the public; groups of women and children were sitting under the fine old trees, and the deer were so tame that they took no notice of passers-by. We sailed up the river to Waterloo Bridge, passing the Tower and St. Paul's, and several handsome stone bridges. Then we went over the British Museum, which is thrown open to the public. We had only time to pass rapidly through hall after hall devoted to branches of natural science, Egyptian monuments, Grecian remains, &c., all admirably classified, with a label to every specimen. How I longed that our students, and particularly a certain E. B., could enjoy the great advantage of walking to such an institution, and seeing each object of study actually there in its natural relations! I hastened home to wash and dress, and reached Mrs. X.'s just in time for the seven o'clock dinner. It was a tremendous operation. We sat at table for three hours. I really grew stiff, notwithstanding the champagne I drank. By-the-by, that is the only wine I like; iced champagne is really good. I sat by Sir J. H. at table, and never discovered till I had left that it was actually mother's old friend. He told Charles that he knew my mother, and remembered my face perfectly, having often seen me at church. I regretted exceedingly that I did not know the connection till too late, for I had always liked the kind old gentleman, and he would have seemed to me quite like an old friend. He has been rather unfortunate in money matters lately, and was robbed of all his family jewels by a foreign count and countess whom he was hospitably entertaining. He possesses an old château in France, which he often visits, and gave me his card to use at Boulogne, in case I went that way. The general conversation, however, was stupid, and I really needed our three-mile walk home to wear off its constraining effects. . . .

Thursday morning I visited my first hospital, St. Thomas's, but under rather unpleasant circumstances; indeed, I hesitated whether to go at all. The surgeon to whom I sent my letter of introduction knew nothing about me, thought it was a very indelicate undertaking, and simply sent me a line to one of the nurses, with the request that I would not enter any of the men's wards. I swallowed the indignity, however, and went, feeling very uncomfortable. But to my surprise, after I had been there a little while I was met by Mr. South, the senior surgeon, who had come on purpose to meet me and show me everything—a very kind, rather eccentric man, who paid me the utmost attention, and pointed out everything, even to the everlasting brewhouse of the establishment. In the museum he drew my attention to many noteworthy specimens, such as the aorta tied by Sir Astley Cooper. St. Thomas's is a series of enormous buildings, which is the character of most public institutions here; its income is 30,000*l*. per annum, and some hospitals have even more. Then he invited me to attend his clinical lecture; so at the head of a large body of students, who had been peeping at me in every direction, I passed with him through ward after ward, men's and women's, the students preserving the most perfect order, though I could see that they were filled with the intensest curiosity. He gave me the fullest description of interesting cases, and made me examine several. He left his students to the house-surgeon, and accompanied me to the Barclay Brewery—an enormous affair, quite a national curiosity. It was here that the brutal Haynau, whilst visiting the place a short time ago, was mobbed by the men when they heard who had come amongst them, and barely escaped some very rough usage. My courteous escort left me in the kindliest manner, promising me an introduction to the Bethlehem. While at St. Thomas's I received three invitations to *post-mortems*, to a lecture, and to the Ophthalmic Dispensary, all of which I was compelled to decline for want of time.

At the brewery visitors enter their names. I set mine down without the M.D.; Mr. South insisted on my adding it. I have been asked by physicians again and again if they shall call me doctor—they fully recognise my right. I always answer this question in the affirmative, as a matter of principle. I can hardly describe to you the difference of feeling with which I entered and left the hospital. We walked a couple of miles to dine with Mr. and Mrs. Charles T., an elegant household, though without the fetters of fashion; they welcomed me most kindly. My two remaining days will be very busy: I have two or three hospitals to visit and several people to see; indeed, engagement treads upon engagement, so that I've hardly a moment to think. I thought such excitement would have bothered me intensely. It did at first bewilder, but now I've roused myself to meet it and I really enjoy it. I've never had such an experience; I must have walked ten miles a day. I come home sometimes hardly able to move a foot; I wash and dress, and in an hour I'm up again and fresh for as much more—the more I have to do, the more I can. I believe I've never yet begun to call out my power of working.

The girl has just come in with my letters, passport, and papers by the "Europa"—what a good sight! Bless you all ten thousand times! My next letter will probably be from Paris. . . .

. . . I have had a delightful visit to Hampstead, where Dr. Wilkinson lives. He received me at once with the greatest kindness and interest, introduced me to his wife, a very sweet woman, graceful and gentle, and to some very pretty black-eyed children. He was disappointed that my stay was so short; told me I ought certainly to spend a year in London, that the longer he lived in it the more wonderful it seemed to him, that every idea was represented there not by a single individual but by a whole class, and that the societies I might study there would be of great service to me as a means of development. He is a tall, strong man, not handsome, wears spectacles, and has a strong expression of goodness in his face. He took me to see two people who were desirous of making my acquaintance, and showed me all the fine points of view from Hampstead, which truly is a most lovely spot, though only two miles from London. It is a hilly range, looking down on wide undulating country on both sides, with blue hills in the distance—Windsor Castle being distinctly visible twenty miles off. I cannot describe the place; it seems to have built itself in one of Nature's choicest nooks. There is a common covered with golden gorse, broken by little dells in which pretty cottages are nestled, and there are old mansions hidden in noble parks, old walls covered with luxuriant ivy, shady lanes with long avenues of trees and smooth hedges of hawthorn and laurel, fields covered with a rich carpet golden with buttercups and daisies, the cows quietly feeding in a veritable paradise to them. Then there are all manner of odd corners and irregular clusters of houses, but everywhere the most intense vegetation. The little cottage occupied by Byron, who used often to resort to this lovely spot, was pointed out to me, and Harrow, where he went to school. We had much interesting conversation. In the omnibus I parted from the doctor with real regret, but quite refreshed by the cordial intercourse.

Journey to Paris.—All my teachers and medical friends in America had strongly advised my going to Paris, as the one place where I should be able to find unlimited opportunities for study in any branch of the medical art. Being then desirous of pursuing surgery as well as medicine, I followed their advice. On May 21, 1849, with a very slender purse and few introductions of any value, I found myself in the unknown world of Paris, bent upon the one object of pursuing my studies, with no idea of the fierce political passions then smouldering amongst the people, nor with any fear of the cholera which was then threatening an epidemic.

Curious glimpses of this outer world are given in letters sent home at that time.

Paris, 11 Rue de Seine: May 1849.

You see, dear friends, that I have reached my destination at last, and fairly established myself in this strange city. I parted from my kind companion, who in London had spent the whole week in one continued effort to aid me in every possible way, with real gratitude. I could not thank him, words seemed too meaningless. . . . I left London with the profoundest respect for the vast power of many kinds displayed there, and a grateful remembrance of a personal reception that had been so encouraging. It rained the whole way over. An English lady returning to Paris with her husband was very friendly. She promised to show me the best place to stay at in Calais, and said if I would travel with them in the cars she could give me much information about Paris, for the French made a point of cheating the English unmercifully, thinking they were immensely wealthy. We were notified of our approach to Calais by a strong smell of fish. It was quite dark and raining in torrents; I was very glad to have companions. We picked our way as well as we could over the stone pier, enclosed by walls on which stood a lighthouse glaring into the dark night. We stepped into the rooms where the passports are examined, and there the whiskered faces showed me I was amongst strangers, and the *Où allez-vous, madame?* confirmed the fact. Next morning I stood for some time on the pier waiting for the Custom-house officer and watching the strange people. Market-women in their white caps (the common people wear no bonnet), groups of workmen in blue blouses, fishwomen of enormous muscular development, though short, returning from fishing laden with their nets, clad in a single petticoat scarcely reaching to the knee, little children with their schoolbooks making sundry excursions on to the fishing-smacks by the way, and chattering French with all their might. At the Custom-house the search was very slight; they did not even see the cases which I had put at the back of a larger trunk, and I was only charged a couple of francs.

We left Calais at nine o'clock, and the difference between France and England was apparent the whole way. The country was no flatter than between Liverpool and Birmingham, but badly drained and badly cultivated, with many peat bogs and dwarf willows bordering the watercourses. There were many villages built of light-coloured stone, but apparently not one brisk, thriving town. The whole way wooden fences instead of beautiful live hedges, women digging trenches and working in the peat bogs, and the railroad left in the rough, unfinished style of America, without the excuse of an immense young country. At the Custom-house in Paris, where they search the trunks for butter and cheese, I parted from my travelling companions and launched boldly into the sea of Paris. It looked very odd as I drove along; the streets so narrow, with such odd, old-fashioned houses, all built of this light-coloured stone, which has no sort of expression. They charged extravagantly at the hotel where I passed the night, so I determined at once to procure lodgings, and set off early next morning to hunt up Mr. Doherty, who I knew through Dr. Wilkinson would tell me the right quarter for medical doings.

I started off with a map in my hand and hope in my heart, and reached Mr. Doherty's house very early, I suppose, for Parisian hours, for the gentleman was in bed when my letters were handed in; and soon after a short sleepy-looking man made his appearance, with a horrid coarse beard, a blue and red woollen dressing-gown, and green baize trousers hanging about his ankles. I had some difficulty in making him comprehend that I was not Anna. At last, however, with the help of letters and my explanations, all became clear. I found him very pleasant; he breakfasted, dressed, &c., while I talked to his brother Thomas, who is a beautiful artist. Mr. D. went with me to some places he knew of. At last we found a little room with bedroom attached in a central situation and at a moderate rent. The hostess was a very pleasant-looking woman, with her own room close by, the whole suite being separated from the rest of the house. I felt, however, quite disappointed in the city; it did not seem to me handsome, gay, or elegant after London; but then, in truth, I was so busy settling my own little matters that I hardly had time to examine closely. Today I have spent in walking about the city with my hostess, chiefly for the sake of chattering with her and accustoming my ear to the strange sounds, for I find I have much to learn. I have great trouble in expressing myself with any elegance, and I cannot see the physicians until I have acquired a tolerable command of words; I shall very soon, however, be able to do so. I went out to buy a bonnet to-day, but found that my unfortunate organs were totally unable to squeeze themselves into a Parisian head-dress; so I was obliged to order a bonnet, choosing plain grey silk, although I was assured again and again that nobody wore that colour. . . .

An interview with Lamartine.—At this period much sympathy was felt in America for the Republican movement in France, of which Lamartine was the head. Before leaving Philadelphia a friend had asked me to be the bearer of one of those expressions of sympathy the public meetings which were then sent to the poet from all parts of the United States. I willingly undertook the commission, and now wrote to the President for permission to present the document entrusted to me.

May 31, 1849.

I have just returned from my visit by appointment to Lamartine, where I went to deliver the Philadelphia resolution entrusted to me. I must hasten to give you a sketch before this post—the last—closes.

Of course I dressed with great care, and arrived just at the appointed hour. I was asked if I was a lady from America, for Lamartine is to most people *in the country*. I was shown through several antechambers into a drawing-room, where stood the poet entertaining some visitors; he bowed, requested me to wait a few moments, and withdrew with his visitors into another room. I examined the apartment; a lofty room, carved and richly gilded, three long windows opening on to a balcony commanding a garden full of trees. The room contained a rich carpet and purple velvet couches and chairs, some portraits, an exquisite female profile in bas-relief, a golden chandelier from the ceiling, some antique vases, &c., and a soft green light from the trees of the large garden diffused through the room. The door opened and Lamartine entered; very tall and slender, but the most graceful man I have ever seen, every movement was music; grey eyes and hair. The little bust is a pretty good likeness. He has the gentlemanly voice (Uncle Charle's), clear, melodious, perfectly well-bred. In fact, his exterior harmonised perfectly with his poetry. He asked me if the resolution referred to the fraternity of the race, and it seemed to understand at once the whole matter when I replied in the affirmative. I referred him to the letters accompanying the resolution for full explanation respecting the document and the manner of presenting it. He said he was very happy to receive these expressions of sympathy. He would read the letters carefully and send me an answer, which I promised to transmit to America. He accompanied me very politely to the stairs, bowed, and we parted. I was so in no way disappointed; there was perfect harmony in the man and his surroundings. Doubtless he is a true man, though unable to work into practice the great thoughts he cherishes.

I went last night with my good little hostess to a neighbouring church, where there is service every evening. It was well lighted round the central altar, but in every direction the lofty aisles stretched away into the darkness, with an occasional lamp illuminating some saint, and small groups of dark figures kneeling on the pavement. The people were assembled in the centre—mostly the lower classes, women in their white caps, and little children dressed like miniature women; they knelt or stood, or sat on chairs and benches as the service required, generally with the utmost devotion. The little children used the holy water, crossed themselves, and knelt with their mothers, and regarded the bright lights, the flowers round the golden Virgin, and the impressive music with eager, wondering faces. The service was sung or chanted entirely in Latin; occasionally a pause in the music would be broken by the sudden, deep tones of a man's voice away in the darkness, or a choir of boys' voices would burst forth apparently from the clouds. The walls were covered with enormous pictures partially illuminated. I felt fully the impressiveness of this scene to the uneducated people; no thought awakened, but the emotional religious sentiment powerfully addressed; and this every night, when the solemn ceremonial contrasts so strongly and soothingly with the traffic of the day. The children are nursed in this atmosphere until it becomes a part of their nature that no reasoning can ever change.

My first introduction to Paris institutions was through the visit of a public official, who brought a registration paper to be filled up. I put myself down as *Etudiante*. The man stared, and then standing in front of me began to make the most extraordinary grimaces, opening his eyes until the whites showed all round them. My first astonished thought was—"You ugly little brute, what on earth are you doing that for?" when, his manner suddenly changing on my look of astonishment, he tapped me benevolently on the shoulder, saying, "*Mon enfant*, you must not put yourself down as student—*rentière* is the word you must use!"

In later life, with larger experience, I came to the conclusion that I had been interviewed by the Police des Mœurs! Fortunately at that time I knew nothing of the corrupt system of accepting and regulating female vice.

My next important interview was of a very different character. A Boston friend had procured for me, from a physician, an introduction to the famous Louis, then at the height of his reputation. It was a sealed introduction, which I forwarded with my card. The next day a tall, imposing-looking gentleman called upon me, who proved to be Louis himself. I soon felt instinctively that his visit was one of inspection. I told him frankly of my earnest desire for hospital and practical instruction. After a long conversation he most strongly advised me to enter La Maternité, where in one most important branch I could in a short time obtain more valuable practical knowledge than could be obtained anywhere else, and he informed me of the steps to be taken in order to obtain admission. Before leaving, however, M. Louis handed to me the letter of introduction which I had sent to him, saying that he thought I ought to see it. It was an astounding production, written in such wretched French that I could only suppose that its author was unaware of its insulting character, or of the effect that such a letter delivered to a French gentleman by a young unknown woman was likely to produce. I never again presented a sealed letter of introduction. Some years later, when the distinguished physician who had sent it called upon me in New York, I returned the letter to him, with a few words of very serious remonstrance.

On June 1 one of my sisters and a friend came to Paris, and we moved into pleasant lodgings in the Rue de Fleurus overlooking the Luxembourg Garden. Whilst there I attended lectures at the Collège de France and the Jardin des Plantes, and earnestly sought for admission to some of the hospitals for practical instruction. It seemed, however, that an entrance into La Maternité would be the most direct first step in obtaining the practical instruction needed, and although regretting the delay in my surgical studies which would be involved in such a course, I finally resolved to pursue the courses of that great institution.

The following letters refer to this period of effort.

MY DEAR COUSIN.—I find that I cannot enter the Maternité at present for want of an *acte de naissance*. I am trying to get over the difficulty, but French regulations are so strict that it is still uncertain whether I can succeed. Would it be possible to secure in Bristol a copy of my register of baptism, with a statement of my birthday and my parents, certified by the mayor or some proper authority? I was baptised at Bridge Street by Mr. Leifchild; I was born on February 3, 1821. I do not know, however, whether such a register is kept in England. If it could be procured, it would remove the difficulty which lies in my way.

We find Paris a very lively residence; every day something new is occurring, or we discover some wonderful old place which we must certainly visit. One day it is the funeral celebrations of Marshal Bugeaud, at which all the great men assist, with an army of soldiers and an enormous crowd; or a thousand little girls take their first communion at St. Sulpice, dressed in white with long veils; or some grand collection of flowers or manufactured articles calls out the spectacle-loving people. There is a constant effervescence of life in this great city, which concentrates all its energy in itself, and makes the Parisians at the same time the most brilliant and the most conceited people in the world. The greatest pleasure which we have yet enjoyed was our trip last Sunday to Versailles; it is really a place to be proud of, and I could not wonder at the worship which is paid to that beautiful temple by the people who, day after day, range freely through its grand galleries and spacious gardens.

I received to-day a very pleasant letter from Dr. Webster, one of our professors at Geneva; I was much gratified to find that their course to me has been approved by the profession in America. It would have grieved me inexpressibly if they had been condemned for the aid they had given me, and there seemed to be some possibility of it when I left. But he tells me my thesis was commented on in the Report on Medicine at the National Medical Convention held in Boston, and their course in relation to me justified and approved. The thesis was received with applause. This information is quite a relief to me, for the thought would be too painful that you could injure your friends.

June 15.

DEAR COUSIN,—By the first of July, as soon as I have conquered some miserable little difficulties, such as the *acte de naissance*, certificate of vaccination, &c., which I cannot produce, I shall enter La Maternité, a world-famous institution, and remain until I have succeeded in my first object—viz. to become an accomplished obstetrician. There are personal objections connected with this course that I was not prepared for—viz. a strict imprisonment, very poor lodging and food, some rather menial services, and the loss of three or four nights' sleep every week. Still, these are things that can be borne (if the health will stand them) when the end to be gained is an important one; and I am sure you will agree with me that it is wise to sacrifice physical comfort for a while in order to attain it. I propose to remain there three months, and then I shall try and accomplish my second object—viz. surgery.

I hope in a day or two to receive permission from the Directeur-General, M. Davenne, to examine all the hospitals of Paris. I am working on gradually; but I find more clearly every day that the genius of the French nation does not suit me, and my love for the Anglo-Saxon race, and my admiration for our wonderful Fatherland, increase by the comparison. . . .

We have had a strange glimpse of a revolution, a sort of theatrical representation of what that terrible thing might be. I confess that the whole exhibition seemed to me peculiarly French; and yet there are noble and terrible passions, lying below this mercurial excitability, that command hearty sympathy or serious consideration, and the unjust, tyrannical acts of the Government excite one's strongest indignation. Now all is quiet again, however, and the whole affair is said to have been planned by the authorities to get rid of certain troublsome men.

A. and E. have stood the shock well, though they turned quite pale on finding as they were quietly parading the streets that they were in the midst of an *émeute*, and later I was sent out to see if they had not better instantly return to England, before civil war broke out and their throats were cut. . . .

On the afternoon of the 13th E. and I went out to see the curious sight. The Quai to the National Assembly, more than a mile long, was lined with soldiers with their drawn bayonets. The Louvre and the Tuileries opposite were closed and filled with soldiers. An army of cavalry was mounted and ready to start at any moment. We passed through hurrying crowds full of excitement, hearing fearful reports of what had happened and what was to come. On the bridges, at the corners of the streets, were large groups of blouses, students, citizens, women, listening to some orator of the moment, gesticulating violently. More than once I observed a woman enthusiastically haranguing an audience. The most curious mixture of passions was visible on the faces—fear, anger, indignation, hope, hatred; there was many a figure that realised the horrors of an earlier revolution. It seems inconceivable now that those violent expressions should have died away, and that Paris is going on in its usual busy way.

June 1849.

MY FRIENDS, ONE AND ALL,—I closed my last letter apparently on the eve of a great insurrection. I went out with E. G. quickly to put it in the post, not knowing how soon we might be prisoners in the house or stirring out at the risk of life. We passed through hurrying crowds full of excitement. Through the night heavy waggons of ammunition and provisions, escorted by soldiers, had rumbled through the streets. The public squares were shut and filled with soldiers. The Democratic press was destroyed; and the next morning the city was declared in a state of siege, and a proclamation was published by the President calling on all good citizens to maintain the authority of the law.

But nothing occurred, the commotion subsided, and the Conservative press congratulated the country on its preservation from the dangerous conspiracy of a few seditious demagogues.

It is difficult to get at the truth in a country where everybody lies upon principle; but it is now commonly believed that the whole affair was a trick of the Government to get rid of Ledru Rollin, Considérant, and other troublesome members of the Montagne, who were determined to call the President to account for his infamous conduct to the poor Romans.

I do not know whether American papers give these particulars—you must tell me if I repeat what you can get better elsewhere—but we have taken deep interest in these events passing round us. Our indignation is much roused against the Conservative tyranny; and the belief in the Government trick shows, curiously enough, of what it may be capable.

A manifestation meeting was called, to support by general feeling the attack which had been made by the advanced party in the Assembly on the unconstitutional measures of the President in suppressing popular gatherings. Two hundred thousand men were passing quietly to the place of meeting, some of the most respectable and distinguished citizens of Paris amongst them, not the slightest disturbance, not even one "Vive la Constitution!" was heard; but a proclamation had been stuck about the streets, of the most inflammatory character, calling the citizens to arms, and signed by Considérant and Ledru Rollin. On the strength of that proclamation, which is fully believed to have been a forgery, the "meeting" was dispersed and proceedings instituted against the members. The Government is proceeding with a high hand. I see that to-day even the Conservative press is putting in a feeble protest.

You would be amused to see how universally politics are discussed: the boy who arranged our rooms, the market-women at their stalls, everyone finds time to read a journal and give some opinion about it.

On June 30 I entered La Maternité; my residence there was an invaluable one at that stage of the medical campaign, when no hospitals, dispensaries, or practical *cliniques* were open to women. La Maternité was a great State institution, where young women to be trained as midwives were sent up from every department of France. The system of instruction, both theoretical and practical, was a remarkable illustration of that genius for organisation which belongs to the French. Every moment of time was appropriated; no distraction of books, newspapers, or other than medical works were allowed; lectures, wardwork, drills, and *cliniques* were arranged from morning to night with no confusion, but no pause; and the comprehension and progress of each pupil was constantly tested by examination.

The institution occupied the old convent of Port Royal, and the discipline was monastic in simplicity, regularity, and seclusion.

Stirring events were occurring in Paris during my residence in the Maternité, but only vague rumours reached us, as no newspapers were allowed within the old grey convent walls.

The following letters give curious pictures of life in this remarkable French institution.

July 1, 1849: à la Maternité.

Dear Mother,—I have now entered upon a strange phase of life, which I must try and describe, that you may imagine me running about in my great white apron, in which respectable article of apparel I expect to figure for the next three months. I had a good many obstacles to encounter from my ignorance of French customs; and the physicians of Paris, as far as I can judge, are determined not to grant the slightest favour to a feminine M.D. I could not obtain from any persons connected with the Maternité the smallest modification to suit the very different status with which I enter from the young French *sages-femmes*; but I was determined to enter on whatever conditions, and enter, too, by the first of July, to habituate myself a little to the ways of the place before the annual lectures commenced. I find now that nothing would have been easier than to have given me a little room to myself, permission to go out occasionally, and similar favours, which need have occasioned no jealousy or inconvenience; for the very fact of my being a foreigner impresses the French girls, and they would freely have accepted any claim made for me. But everything was obstinately refused to all the representations of myself or the Consul, Mr. Walsh, and I was only too glad to enter as a young, ignorant French girl. On June 30 I drove, down with Anna to the hospital. A high stone wall, with the tops of old buildings peeping above, extends nearly the whole length of a little street. A very small door led into a dark little entrance, the *portiére* on one side, and a long room, called by courtesy the *parloir*, on the other. You must notice the *parloir*, for it is there I shall receive my visitors, if I ever have any, at two o'clock, in common with the other *élèves*; and there in one corner, in a sort of little glass box, sits the good dame who attends to the letters and transacts all the outdoor business for the *élèves*. The ceiling is very low, the floor of brick, rows of wooden benches ranged one before the other—the most uninteresting room you can possibly conceive; the only pretty thing being the vine leaves which peep through the diamond-shaped windows. This room forms part of a row of old buildings standing against the wall, which contain the director's bureau, the *Interne's* rooms, &c. It was too late for me to see M. Boivin, the director, so an old woman took me into the central buildings, through a labyrinth of little passages and long galleries, and all manner of rooms and queer places, to Madame Charrier, the *sage-femme* in chief, who has her own rooms in a particular part of the building. Her parlour is the funniest little cabinet of curiosities, with a carpet on the floor, as it is of brick instead of waxed wood. Little chintz sofas, mosaic tables, boxes, china and figures, crucifixes, pictures and embroideries, and curtains everywhere, Madame Charrier is a little deformed woman, elderly, but with a fresh colour still, and kind blue eyes. I like what I have seen of her; she seems generally loved by the pupils, and though I do not imagine her of any particular amount of intellect, she seems to have good sense, and after twelve years in such an establishment as this she ought to have much valuable experience. Madame Charrier conducted me by unknown ways to Madame Blockel, the superintendent of the *dortoirs*, who took me into the infirmary, and said I must sleep there until I had arranged my affairs with the director. I did not much admire the idea of passing the night in the infirmary. There was a large wood fire on the hearth, and the air felt warm and somewhat close. I looked suspiciously at the long rows of beds extending on each side, their white curtains closely drawn; I did not know what undesirable emanations might be proceeding from them. However, I said nothing, but determined to investigate the contents of the beds as soon as the observers had withdrawn. My trunk was brought up, my bed pointed out, a little lamp placed on the table, and I was left alone. I proceeded then to make my observations, and found to my great relief that every bed was empty, except one, in which one of the *élèves*, who happened to have a headache, was lying, and from her I found that the place is healthy and no epidemic has prevailed there for a long time. I found her, like all the other French girls, full of those light kindnesses which are so pleasant. She asked me eagerly if I was from her province, and seemed to regard me with much interest when she found I was a stranger from New York, which was the only part of the United States she had heard of, and which she took to be an island near Havannah. I have since found that the pupils are much disappointed that I am not black, as they supposed all persons from America were! After talking a little with her I took out my writing materials, and sat down to the table determining to pay a little visit across the water before going to rest in my new home; but I had no sooner seated myself than Madame Charrier entered with a crowd of *élèves*, to know if I would pass the night in the *salle d'accouchements*, it being an optional matter the first night. Of course I expressed the utmost willingness. I put up my letter with a sigh, dressed myself for duty, and accompanied an *ancienne élèves* (that is, one who has already studied a year, and who always has one or more of the *nouvelles élève* under her care for initiation) to the room where the children are born. A large apron of coarse towelling was given me, with the injunction not to lose it, or I should have to pay three francs. It was a large upper room, rather dimly lighted, beds all round, a fire on the hearth, cupboards full of linen in the corners, heaps of shining copper and tin utensils, several rush-bottomed chairs and wooden tables, and in the centre a large wooden stand with sides, on which the little new-comers, tightly swathed and ticketed, are ranged side by side. In the course of the night we had the pleasure of arranging *eight* in this way, and the next morning when Madame Charrier made her appearance the cloth was removed and the sight shown with much triumph. It was really very droll. Each little shapeless red visage peeped from under a coarse peaked cap, on the front of which was a large label with the name and sex; a black serge jacket with a white handkerchief pinned across, and a small blanket tightly folded round the rest of the body, completed the appearance of the little mummy. Their behaviour certainly realised

Fourier's supposition, for there was very little crying all the time they lay there together. There were four young French girls sitting up with me, besides the girl who makes the beds and does the roughest work. They were all pretty and pleasant, of no education except their studies in the institution; but those had been evidently carefully attended to, and it sounded not a little droll to hear the scientific terms flowing so glibly from their laughing lips, which were busily employed in talking nonsense all the time that their duties did not call them to the bed-side. The next morning at ten o'clock we were discharged from duty; it was Sunday, a comparatively leisure day, and I being a Protestant was excused from the religious services, but I was too sleepy to do much. I wrote, walked in the garden and read a little there, retired early, and had a most welcome sleep and very pleasant dreams.

Our *dortoir* is a large airy room, with a row of windows and beds on each side, divided into two by a large archway; it contains sixteen beds, occupied mostly by *anciennes élèves*. I have a window behind my bed; I have shoved the bed forward, fitted in a chair behind, hung up my dressing-gown, and put a few books on the floor by my side, and call it my room. I am now sitting there writing to you. I have just room enough to move my right arm freely, but I am out of the way, I am breathing fresh air, so I consider myself very well off. An old crucifix ornamented by gilded leaves hangs at one end of the *dortoir*, two little lamps are suspended from the ceiling, an iron bedstead and a chair are appropriated to each individual. The floor is formed of little hexagon bricks, which in some of the rooms are so terribly polished that I walk on them with difficulty. The *dortoir* is seldom quiet; the girls sit there a good deal, and some who have watched through the night are generally there in bed; and how French girls do chatter! How they do go into sudden fits of ecstasy or rage! Once at least in the day we have a grand storm, Madame Blockel coming in for some trouble or other, in which she and the accused out-scream each other, and appear to be mortal enemies for a few minutes, and the best of friends immediately after. At twelve o'clock we receive our supply of bread for the day, which we keep in our bedroom and take backwards and forwards to meals. I have frequently wished that you could see me walking gravely along the gallery with my loaf of bread wrapped in a napkin under my arm. The dining-room is a large hall full of round tables, only three of which are occupied at present, as the *élèves* only number thirty, instead of ninety, the usual number. At dinner I saw them all together for the first time; some very pretty and graceful, some very rough. I am learning to take wine; everyone advises me to do so, and I shall soon be able to drink my bottle a day.

There seems to be an admirable organisation of work here in every department. I have been much amused today by the lessons in theory that I have received from my *ancienne élève* or *chef*. The pupils all sat round, and the young instructress, furnished with some bones, gave out an explanatory sentence, which was repeated by each one in turn; I found it an excellent plan of learning French. Of course, the repetition would have been intolerable without the language, but to listen to a dozen different voices and to repeat myself I found to be admirable practice; indeed, being cut off from all English communication is a great advantage in learning French.

July 3.—This morning I finish my letter in another situation. I wrote last night till it was dark, and the little lamp in our *dortoir* gave so much darkness that I went to bed for want of light. To-day I am *en service*—that is to say, I shall spend the day from eight in the morning till eight in the evening in superintending the six rooms of the infirmary. I have been handling leeches for the first time (disgusting little things). I enter with an *ancienne élève*, who shows me all the ways of the house. At present the lectures have not commenced, but the visits of Madame Charrier and the physician take place every day; and nature is always here in great abundance to be studied. I feel I shall gain a great deal, and hitherto it has really not proved nearly so formidable an imprisonment as I supposed. The air is delightful this beautiful summer weather, the girls pleasant. There is much to interest in so large an establishment, and I suppose the three months will soon slip away, for I have entered, in my own mind, only for the three months, though I have been asked so often if I am going to stay two years that I have had to tell a great many—evasions. I shall have, doubtless, many weary moments, but I want you all to know that it will not be so utterly miserable as my former letters may have represented it. And great will be the reward! So send a welcome greeting to the Voluntary Prisoner.

July 1849.

DEAR M.,—I last wrote to you when I was my own mistress; now in some measure I have given up my liberty, and I must give you a little sketch of my prison life, that you may be able to picture the surroundings of your sister M.D. Imagine a large square of old buildings, formerly a convent, set down in the centre of a great court with a wood and garden behind, and many little separate buildings all around, the whole enclosed by very high walls, over the tops of which, shining out beautifully against the clear sky, may be seen the dome of the Pantheon, the Hôtel des Invalides, and the whole building of the observatory which is close adjoining. The inner court is surrounded by *les cloîtres*, a most convenient arched passage which gives covered communication to the whole building, and which I suppose was formerly traversed by shaven monks on their way to the church, whose great painted window looks out into the court, but which now echoes the laughter of many merry girls, and across which at half-past seven every morning you may see your humble servant with her coarse *tablier de service* and little white pot in hand hurrying to get some coffee. At half-past five every morning I start up in bed, roused by the bustle of the *élèves*, who are up before me. I make violent efforts to drive away sleep, which are only partially successful, and then follow the example of twenty girls who inhabit the same long *dortoir*, and who are busy each by her own iron bedstead dressing hastily to be ready for the visit. I hasten upstairs to the long corridor, the "Sainte-Elisabeth," where my patients lie. I inquire carefully their condition, wash them, and see that the beds have been properly arranged. By that time it is a quarter past six; Madame Charrier makes her appearance and goes the rounds, accompanied by the *élèves*, each one giving a short report of the patients under her care. It is a funny group: fifty women or more of all ages, wide awake from the hurry of their duties, but dressed mostly in haste with little white caps, coloured handkerchiefs, and the coarser ones in short bed-gowns, their faces browned by the sun, their hands red with hard work, but all good-tempered, with a kind word always ready, and their black eyes sparkling with life. We pass through the Salles Sainte-Marguerite, Sainte-Elisabeth, Saint-Anne, visiting each patient in her alcove—it is seven when we finish. I hasten back to my *dortoir*, make my bed, &c., fetch my coffee, which I procure for two sous a morning from the superintendent of the infirmary, eat it hastily with my bread, which is always supplied for the day at noon, and then hurry off to the Salles Sainte-Marie and Sainte-Marthe, where the more sick patients are placed, whom the attending physicians visit every morning at eight. At this visit are present M. Girardin, the chief physician, a tall, dry, grey-haired man, full of pomposity; the *interne*, M. Blot, a very handsome, somewhat dignified young physician, with, I fancy, rather a cross temper; Madame Charrier, the *aide-sage-femme*, and as many of the *élèves* as choose to be present. This over, I make some independent visits to cases which interest me, to the nursery, &c., and try to pick up a little here and there; then I return to the *dortoir* and read or write a little. Afterwards I join the class instruction in the wood, a preparatory lesson which the elder *élèves* give to the younger ones, and which I attend for the sake of the French. It is a very pretty method of instruction: the young teacher seated on the grass, all the pupils grouped around under the thick shade of some fine tree, the atmosphere being of an elastic purity which is truly charming. The French girls have a natural talent for instruction; they are so in the habit of talking that they never find the slightest difficulty in expressing what they know, and their lively perceptions give them a perculiar power for superficial instruction. Our poor country girls find it very hard at first to catch scientific words that they do not understand, but in a surprisingly short time they roll them off smoothly and to a certain extent understand well what is taught them.

At twelve the bell sounds for the first meal, only milk being given at seven o'clock. We enter a large hall, full of round tables, each holding twelve; to each are furnished a couple of white plates, a tumbler and small bottle of wine, a loaf of bread, a spoon and fork. The meal consists of soup, boiled meat, and vegetables; it is eaten in haste to the music of Madame Blockel's voice, which keeps up a storm the whole time. She is a somewhat important personage, superintending our meals and our *dortoirs*; she is a little red-faced, squint-eyed being, with tremendous projecting teeth, and dressed always in rusty black with a black cap. She is good-natured, liked by the girls, but has a tremendous vocal organ, which is always sounding forth at its highest pitch. Morning, noon, and night good Madame Blockel's voice drowns all opposing sounds; and really now I am getting as used to it as to a noisy street, and would not care if only she would keep out of the *dortoir* at night when I am sleepy, for, like a barking dog, she sets all the girls going, and I don't know when the storm subsides, for I sink to sleep in spite of it. When the meal is over we present a funny sight, each carrying off her loaf, napkin, knife, and various bottles and remnants of dinner. I return to the *dortoir*, do up little matters, read or attend the class again, visit my patients in the corridor, and from two to three go to the *parloir* to see my friends, if they are so good as to come at that hot hour to see me. This *parloir* is a funny affair—a plain room, filled with wooden benches, where all manner of rough people are assembled to visit the *élèves*. On certain days, also, in one corner a woman establishes a little shop, where she supplies all the small wants of the girls in the way of haberdashery, stationery, perfumery, &c.; and in another corner sits an old lady, *la dame du bureau*, observing everything, and giving the signal precisely at three for the departure of everybody. At six a second meal is served, consisting of roast meat and some little kind of cake, and another bottle of wine; afterwards we are free to do as we choose. I generally sit a little in the wood and write till it is dark; in a few days, however, the lectures commence, and four or five days will be occupied in that way. I have described my idle, or rather my free days. When I am *en service* I spend the whole day in the ward where I am placed; or the night, if I happen to be on night service. About three or four days are thus spent, and after passing the night in watching I am not worth much the next day, for I am not yet accustomed to the duty. Then little extra touches come in to diversify the day. I pay a visit to Madame Charrier or to Mlle. Mallet, one of the *aides-sage-femmes*, whom I like very much, or some difficult operation calls us to the amphitheatre. Next week I shall be able to tell you how I like the lectures; we shall have several each day, and I hope they will supply the want which I now feel of an intelligent explanation of the phenomena which I observe.

August.—The lectures have now commenced. From seven to eight Madame Charrier gives her lesson every morning; I occupy a chair beside her in consideration of my foreignness, she being anxious that I should understand thoroughly. I wish I could describe that lesson to you; it is the most curious spurring-up of pupils I ever saw, and really it makes some of them gallop admirably, though many tumble down in the effort. Three pupils are called down every morning, seated on a long bench in front of Madame Charrier's table, and undergo an hour's examination on what they have heard from the teachers. If they answer promptly and well, her satisfaction is extreme, her face grows beautiful, and her "Bien! très bien!" really does me good, it is so hearty; but if an unlucky pupil hesitate, if she speak too low, if intelligence or attention be wanting, then breaks forth the most admirable scolding I ever listened to. Alternately satirical and furious, she becomes perfectly on fire, rises upon her chair, claps her hands, looks up to heaven, and the next moment, if a good answer has redeemed the fault, all is forgotten, her satisfaction is as great as her anger. There is not the slightest wickedness about her; she puts her whole soul into her lesson, and does not realise how very difficult it is for ignorant girls to study a science. At first I was a little shocked at this stormy instruction, but really it seems almost necessary now, and produces wonderful results. If the girls only keep their temper under it and do not cry, it comes right at last; but a tear is an unpardonable offence, and considered an insult and a total misunderstanding. Madame Charrier is a woman of great experience and always speaks to the point, and her lessons are often very useful. From nine till ten we listen to M. Paul Dubois. I like his lectures exceedingly. A little, bald, grey-haired man, with a clear, gentle voice and a very benevolent face, he thoroughly understands his subject, and expresses himself with precision and completeness.

At a little after twelve our dinner-bell rings, and right glad I always am to hear it. The large round tables are speedily encircled, all stand up, and a grace is said with such rapidity that to this day I can make out no words but *saint usage*, and the sign of the cross made with wonderful dexterity on the forehead and breast. At the conclusion of the meal another prayer rocket is sent up, amidst laughing and bustle, and all crowd out of the hall, with their loaves of bread under their arms and all manner of odd little pots full of eatables in their hands. From one till two another lesson in the amphitheatre—which, fortunately, is a pleasant room—from the second *aide-sage-femme*, a lesson useful on the whole, but sometimes a little wearisome. From two to three is the hour for receiving visitors, but if I am not expecting a visit, and if I have sat up the preceding night, I take a bath—for there are six baths prepared every day at that hour for the *élèves*. The same communism exists in the baths as in everything else. They are side by side, in a double row, down the middle of the room; and the withered genius of the bath-room stands, observing every movement, and talking an incomprehensible *patios* the whole time. I try to imagine it is only the bubbling of water that I hear; I shut my eyes, lie quietly for half an hour, and fancy that I am deliciously reposing on the heaving waters of some soft summer lake; then I spring up, take a cold dash, to the horror of my companions, and hurry off as fast as possible, really the better for the divine element. . . .

Were I a good Catholic I should find my time filled with visits to the chapel—morning and evening prayers, vespers, and the daily baptisms are regular services, with numerous extras on saints' days, &c.; but most happily I am Protestant, and again and again I have blessed Heaven for the fact. The great fat, red-faced priest occasionally leaves the retirement of his clerical dwelling and strolls in the wood, or makes a visit to the infirmary; he always gives me long stares of excessive curiosity when I pass him, but I have taken a great dislike to his sensual-looking worship, and will not give him the slightest opportunity to make my acquaintance. . . .

After dinner, when fine, I generally go into our wood, and, seating myself under my favourite tree, I write till it grows dark; or I stroll up and down the broad alleys, sending my thoughts far off into the past or the future. It is very pleasant in our wood; outside the walls are large gardens and public walks, so that the air is very fresh, and the beauty of the Parisian summer climate is extreme. Sometimes my friendly *aide* joins me, for she cannot bear to see me alone; it seems to the French a sign of deplorable melancholy. She walks with me, chatting gaily, and bearing my clumsy French with great patience; for, as I said, she has taken a fancy to me, and I have to welcome with a good grace the pinches, shakes, and similar tokens of French affection. Fortunately, however, it shows itself in more satisfactory ways also, and I owe many an opportunity for interesting observation to her kindness. The girls look picturesque in the wood by the sunset light. Sometimes a group is seated on the grass round its chief, eagerly taking in the instruction that may aid it in the next day's examination; others are singing or playing; but I think I have never seen one engaged by herself in meditation or work. Their character is eminently social, communicative. Mr. Doherty remarked wisely that vanity, in its widest sense, is their ruling spirit, which makes it impossible for them to understand the English, where pride rules. There is one young girl I like to talk with. I have never seen anything more graceful, lively, and finished than the little pictures of life which she throws off with perfect ease; every motion of her pretty little head, every gesture and intonation is perfect, and occasionally I am really startled by a profound view of life that she just glances at, and then is off again. I would give much to be able to note down some of her narrations, but when I try to turn them into language their exquisite spirit seems to vanish. . . .

You must not be surprised if my letter contains an immense number of perplexed parentheses, and has a tendency to return always to the same subject. If you could only hear "what hideous sounds salute mine ear," you would not wonder. The girls are singing hymns to the Virgin in an adjoining room, and really, if the Virgin be a lady of as much taste as beauty according to the representations of Raphael, she must be considerably annoyed by the zeal without knowledge displayed by her admirers. Our second *aide-sage-femme* is a very pious young Catholic, of really a sweet disposition. A week or two ago, on the commencement of the month of Mary, she assembled the girls together, reminded them of the season, and proposed to meet frequently in the evening and sing canticles in honour of the Lady, adding that undoubtedly the object of their attention would be gratified by this demonstration and would not be unmindful of those who offered the homage. The proposition was received with enthusiasm, and since that unlucky day Mlle. Boisonnet and her followers have exercised their lungs in season and out of season, to the horror of all my nerves and, I fear, to the serious displeasure of the Virgin. They have numerous little books of canticles. I looked over the index the other day—"Who so pure as she," "The brightness of her presence," "Mary, pray for us," and all such titles filled the pages. The tunes have a striking resemblance to American camp-meeting hymns. There is one which was certainly the original of "Oh, let us be joyful." I often think, if H. were only here, how he would join in honouring the Virgin. . . .

I must give you a few more sketches of my present life. Imagine, then, that you have retired early to bed, after a night spent in hard work, and the day in that nervous mystification that follows loss of rest. You have taken a refreshing bath and laid yourself down, encircled by dear memories that fan you to sleep with their gentle dreams; you have just entered that beautiful dreamland, when you are suddenly startled by a scream, a burst of laughter, and then the vision of one white-robed form darting past in the twilight, pursued by a similar form, mysterious to your veiled senses. The chase continues over beds and boxes, while shouts of laughter, followed by a shower of small articles, proceed from the other beds; then a loud smack is heard, whose nature is easily divined by those who are at all familiar with juvenile offenders, a spring from the bed and a rush by the injured party follow; but still you resolutely shut your eyes and will yourself asleep, in the fond hope that nature is really too tired to keep awake, when a sudden rolling sound, followed by a violent shock, at once convinces you of the vanity of your efforts, and you resign yourself to wakefulness, for a favourite amusement has commenced—they are "promenading the bedsteads"! You must know that our bedsteads are of iron, and placed on rollers so movable that a slight impulsion will speed them a considerable distance. Often in stepping into bed the slight movement has caused the mercurial article to describe a sudden semicircle. This property of these usually sober pieces of furniture is taken advantage of by the girls, who are now in a frolic and exercising in the most ingenious way, to the unspeakable annoyance of a quiet individual. An impulsion is given to one end of a long row of beds, which is quickly communicated to the whole row, or a simultaneous shock is given to the two extremities and their force brought to bear on the unfortunate centre. But the favourite freak is to place a bedstead at the end of the room and drive it with great violence down the centre. The rolling noise over the brick floor is tremendous, and accompanied by a regular Babel of laughter, shouting, and jokes of every description. Some get on top of their beds, which consist of three thick mattresses, and jump up and down like mad things; others get up a wild dance in one corner of the room, which grows continually faster and noisier, and the strife of tongues is truly astonishing. Their jokes are really amusing occasionally; the scientific terms that they hear daily play a conspicuous part. The frolic ends as suddenly as it began, when, fairly fully of fun, they suddenly jump into bed, say good-night, and in five minutes all are sound asleep. The first night I was thus rudely awakened I was much inclined to be angry, but I philosophised a little and came to the conclusion that it was my voluntary action to be there, and that youthful spirits must have free play. I pitied the poor children in their undeveloped life and the restrictions they suffer here too much to be disturbed by their little outburst, and the next morning they begged me to excuse them because they were *so young*!

My time is very fully occupied; my former leisure moments are now employed in writing compositions and taking observations. These last I willingly consent to; they will be records to me of French practice. They consist of a little history of the patient and a daily account of her condition and treatment. But as they are in French, I am somewhat longer in noting them down than I should be if I could employ my own noble language. I have made two "observations" of surgical cases that have been very much approved of. I was quite amused with one of them. I was directed to note the case down under the direction of my chief in that department. As usual, I did promptly and cheerfully what was required; I wrote all she dictated, and then I made a private memorandum for my own satisfaction. This latter was seen by the Superior, and immediately the "chief" was directed to copy it; she did it willingly, for she is a good little being, and has a profound respect for the stranger. The other day two of our chiefs begged me to give them a private lesson on the circulation of the blood, which I willingly complied with. We seated ourselves in the wood, and I explained to them what they did not know; they were very grateful, and have come to me several times since to beg me to continue my lesson—indeed, the girls here have a sweet nature in many respects. There are little jealousies and excitements amongst themselves, but they take the right relationship to me; they think me singularly grave and self-sufficing, but they show me continually the utmost respect, and are always glad to do me any little service. I frequently enter the *salle d'accouchements*, when the other divisions are engaged there, to see what is going on, and I always meet a pleasant welcome. One evening I phrenologised them, to their unbounded delight; for some time after I could never enter the room without being surrounded by a small mob eagerly demanding an examination. Everything delights them; they are perfect children in their full, unthinking enjoyment of the present. A little English lesson is a never-failing source of merriment, and I am continually saluted with some oddly pronounced English word, followed by a burst of merriment. We have girls from all parts of France; some are remarkable for their stupidity, which is generally explained by the province from which they arrive. Madame Charrier's morning lesson is an ordeal through which all have to pass, and seated by her, every morning, I have a fine opportunity for studying the various departments of France. When some singularly obtuse intellect has exhausted all the patience and all the impatience of the teacher, she folds her hands and asks in a subdued voice, "Mademoiselle, from what department do you come?" and on receiving the answer, adds, "Ah, then it is all accounted for; the case is a hopeless one"; which announcement greatly delights the rest of the class who belong to more enlightened departments.

We have one *élève* who goes by the name of "La Normande"; she is one of my *pictures*. A fresh, healthy complexion, browned by the sun and the sea air of her beautiful home, regular features, a stout, vigorous frame that has never known a touch of sickness, she walks about with a step that feels the ground; in her white quilled cap, and handkerchief pinned over her bosom, she looks with her clear blue eyes right into your face, and has a frank, loyal manner that marks her honest, independent nature. On Sunday she dresses in the short full petticoat, the silk-laced jacket, and the lace cap, with its towering pyramidal crown and circular ray-like border, that I think I have already described to you. She sometimes visits our *dortoir* and forms the centre of a group, whom she entertains with her constantly overflowing life, sometimes singing, in a deep contralto voice, her peasant hymns to the Virgin—simple pathetic melodies chanted under the lindens when the day's labours are finished—or dancing vigorously the figures, more gay than graceful, of her country, while she sings some lively air. I admire her vigorous life, I like to see her in the infirmary; she tends the sick with such an honest awkwardness, such a kind heart, and lifts them like babies in her strong arms, that I see the green fields and smell the sweet country air as I watch her. Then I have a little Parisian that I hang up beside her, as plump as a partridge, with merry black eyes, glossy hair always arranged *à la mode*, and full of little coquettish ways. Her temper is like a lucifer match, the slightest friction fires it; the smile and the tear are equally ready, though the sunshine generally prevails. She has spent several years in business in Paris, in cigar stores and similar employments, where she has had much to do with gentlemen, and she repeats to me the compliments they paid her, the offers they made, and her own witty, contemptous replies, with the utmost *naïveté*. Poor child! she has been thrown on her own simple instincts for protection, for her mother was soon jealous of the attractions of her daughter, and removed her to a distance; but the real innoncence of her heart, and a true attachment to a young ship's surgeon, seem to have supplied the place of her natural protectors. But true to her Parisian blood, she has coquetted from first to last, and she never talks to me now but I find it playing in every dimple. Think of it! she was given me as my "Chief of Theory"! Now she asks me in the sweetest manner if I will come sometimes to her lessons, and explain to the girls what she does not understand. Poor child! I willingly oblige her.

But I must not weary you with my portrait gallery, my walls are covered with curious figures; let me sketch for you our "vaccinations," which take place every Tuesday at one o'clock. The numbers of the babies are distributed beforehand amongst the *élèves* who are to perform the operations; thus, 25 Ste. Marie to one, 32 Ste. Marthe to another, and so on. The *élèves* seek their babies and bring them into the Hall of the Nurses, a large upper room, full already of women and babies. A space is cleared by one of the windows, chairs placed; in the centre sits M. Blot, the director of the operation; I occupy a chair beside him. Mademoiselle, who superintends another division, stands beside, and then baby after baby is subjected to the awkward manœuvres of the *élèves*, to their utmost dissatisfaction. The babies are very ugly in their coarse hospital swaddling clothes; I never saw the little beings so enveloped before. They are just like mummies, but they perform a terrible concert altogether, with the voices of the *élèves* to help them. I sit a quiet spectator of the operation, occasionally addressing a question to M. Blot as he touches knife after knife on the arm of the infant before him; which question seems rather to embarrass the handsome *interne*, for he colours, or passes his hand through his hair and looks intently at the baby, in a very un-Frenchmanlike manner. I think he must be very *young*, or very much in awe of me, for he never ventures to give me a direct look, and seems so troubled when I address him that I very rarely disturb his life in that way.

I think I have given you enough of my external hospital life to enable you to picture me somewhat in my surroundings; do you want to know how the spirit feels in its curious home? Then know, dear friends, that it is strong and hopeful, that it has moments of weariness, of intense yearning for its true related life, but that it lives ever in the great presence of the Eternal, and feels the angels always near.

The difficult breaking-in to the practical work of the obstetrician is noted in the journal of those days; and also the pleasant comradeship which gradually sprang up with the very intelligent young physician who served as *interne* at that time; this companionship was a great relief to my imprisonment in La Maternité.

NOTES FROM THE JOURNAL

July 4.—Attended lessons by the *aides-sages-femmes*; very clever instruction. Spent the day in the *salle d'accouchements*, but was disgusted by the treatment of a *primipara*. With all the instruction they have received, the very first principles of humane treatment seem too often neglected. They are still ignorant midwives with their mischievous interference. . . . The version seemed to me horrible. I almost fainted. . . . Spent the night in the infirmary—weary work. I cannot bear this loss of sleep. . . . To-day, three operations; much interested in the morning, but grew weary and disgusted in the afternoon.

July 22.—Attended the *interne's* visit and spoke to him about one of the patients; he replied so pleasantly that I said a little more, and he promised to lend me a medical journal to look over, and see how I liked it. The little friendliness encouraged me. . . .

August 12.—The poor woman whom I have attended as my first complete patient gave me a little *prie-dieu* which she had made. Her humble heart longs to express its gratitude. I put it in my Bible where my friends are reading to-day. . . . M. Dubois again waited after the lecture to say a few pleasant words. He wished I would stay a year and gain the gold medal; said I should be the best obstetrician, male or female, in America! Had quite a pleasant visit to the infirmary, where M. Blot made me observe several interesting points, and answered my questions intelligently and frankly. . . .

August 24.—Quite taken by surprise at the infirmary visit this afternoon. M. Blot met me so pleasantly, and asked me to give him some lessons in English. I think he must have been meditating this request for some time; it had hardly the air of a spontaneous thought. I like him. I hope we may come a little more closely together. . . .

September 2.—I have been quite happy for three hours. I must note down what I've learned. M. Blot brought his microscope to the Infirmerie des Élèves. I was exceedingly interested in his microscopic lecture. He showed us in a work of M. Hébert's the difference between the epithélium pavimenteux, such as covers the tongue, skin, &c., and the epithélium vibratile, as in other parts, and the fibro-plastic formations in the reparation of tissues, showing specimens of each kind. The first species was represented by a cellule full of little cellules, a *noyau* in the centre containing a nucleolus—thus. . . . The second was of elongated form, thus. . . . The third represented the growth of fibre, from cells, which cells are distinguished from the first by the relatively smaller size of the *noyau*, thus. . . . By such examination different formations can be distinguished from each other; thus cancer possesses very distinctive elements. It is necessary to examine bodies of varying shapes under different foci of the microscope, otherwise illusions may be created. In illustration he placed some blood globules, and showed us that what appeared a central spot in each globule was owing to the convexity not being in focus, and it disappeared when the focus was a little lengthened. He spoke also of a paper read before a society yesterday by a young physician, which proved that the azote, which in the ox is voided by the excrement, in the cow is absorbed into the milk; and that the difference in the manure of the two is great.

He is busy himself now in preparing for an examination of *internes*; if he gain the gold medal, he has the right to enter any hospital he chooses as *interne* for a second term, and receive also his M.D., not otherwise granted to an *interne*. What chance have women, shut out from these instructions? Work on, Elizabeth! . . .

To-day M. Blot spoke of a friend, Claude Bernard, a distinguished young inquirer, who is now, he thinks, on the eve of a discovery that will immortalise him—viz. the discovery of an accessory circulation, by which substances are sent directly to the kidneys without traversing the general circulation, which will explain, for instance, the rapid effect of champagne on the kidneys. This second heart is situated in the ascending vena cava, close by the liver; strong muscular fibres are evident in the human subject, but in the horse are as large as quills. He does not perceive yet what veins return the blood, if his supposition be true. He also spoke of the power which the liver has of secreting sugar in a normal state, when animals are fed on certain substances which can be so converted; also of the curious experiment by which a dog was made, in his presence, to secrete albuminous or diabetic urine, according to the pricking of one or another point of the pneumogastric nerve near its origin. . . .[1]

At the afternoon visit we had quite a philosophical discussion on society, &c. Mlle. Mallet was delighted with a *bon mot* of M. Blot. She remarked that she understood that *les demoiselles* had answered like *anges*. "Yes," he answered, "*en ôtant le g*." They had been unusually

1. I was at that time utterly unaware of the amount of degrading cruelty perpetrated by many foreign investigators upon helpless animals under methods erroneously called scientific. It required the extended observation of the physician to realise the intellectual fallacy necessarily involved in experiments which destroy the thing to be observed; and also to recognise how the constant promulgation of false theory and practice arising from erroneous methods of investigation hinders the attainment of scientific medicine.

I have long since realised that conscience and humanity must guide intellectual activity and curiosity, or we wander from the highroad of truth into a labyrinth of error. The above experience illustrates how the eager young student, thirsting for knowledge, may be blind to the unscientific or immoral methods of pseudo-science.

stupid! She asked me if M. Blot were not rather *moqueur.* I said I did not know, but that I had discovered that he was very ambitious. His sentiments seem to be good, but his character is certainly not French.

September 21.—M. Dubois stopped to speak to me after the lecture, and again expressed his great desire that I should remain a year in the institution. I told him I had determined to remain another three months; but I had many other branches to study. He replied that anything else I might learn elsewhere as well as in Paris, but that the opportunity of seeing all that was remarkable in three thousand deliveries in that space of time could be met with nowhere else in the world; that it equalled the whole practice of most physicians, and he was persuaded that I should regret it if I did not remain. He parted saying he would talk the matter over again with me. If it be pure interest that makes him urge this, I am glad; but it seems to me now an impossible endurance.

October 4.—Another midnight scene—a strange spectacle of suffering and of science. As I stood on the crowded benches of the amphitheatre I heard the clock strike one, the holy noon of night. I wondered how long our sins would thus be fearfully visited upon us. The rain beat in torrents on the skylight, the wind shook the building, and I could look with intense interest on that rare and dangerous accident submitted to our investigation—lithotomy, the only way to save life; a tedious operation lasting, I should think, an hour, for in the hurry of midnight dressing I had forgotten my watch. . . .

To-night I have been walking in the wood; the wind blows fresh under the clear starlight. I am happier now that my mind is clearly determined to leave at the end of six months, with the conviction that my work here is thoroughly done. . . .

October 30.—Madame Charrier sent for me this afternoon to present me with *my portrait.* It was a lithograph picture of Elizabeth Blackwell, taken from a history of *sages-fammes célèbres.* This lady, about 1737, published a work on medical botany in two large folio volumes, in order to get her husband, a medical man, out of prison, where he was confined for debt.

I imagined a whole romance out of the picture, and a little biography—a romance of a beautiful, true spirit, struggling with a society too strong to be turned from its ancient habits of evil. But the pure spirit is not lost, it is working bravely still.

A SORTIE FROM LA MATERNITÉ

October 22.

Dear Friends, One and All,—Yesterday I spent a delightful day—a day which I passed in doing nothing—and it was so pleasant, so refreshing, that I must tell you about it. I had laid out so many plans for my first day of freedom. I was to see so many medical people, and so many medical places, that I was almost exhausted in the aniticipation, and when my leave of absence actually came, when all things worked right, and I was neither *en service*, nor in the infirmary, nor in the reception, and when moreover, for a wonder, it did not rain, I just determined to give up everything like business, forget there was such a thing as medicine or such a place as the Maternité, and give myself up like a child to the pleasure of looking and moving and eating, and everything that was natural and nothing that was wise! In fact, I found that I could really do nothing of business in a satisfactory way in the short space of eleven hours, so my troublesome conscience for once was quiet, and permitted me to waste a day. I was really amused at myself to find how anxious I was that it should not rain, and how impatient I was for the moment to arrive when I could leave, for by the rules of the place Anna must take me out, and Anna must bring me back precisely at eight o'clock! The *directeur* could not help laughing when he informed me of these regulations; still, as he said, "no exceptions could be made." Anna was anxious that I should lose no portion of my short day. She woke up an hour earlier than usual, with the sense of some weighty responsibility resting upon her, which she could not at first understand; but as the idea of the Maternité dawned upon her she rose in haste, and at nine o'clock the summons for Mademoiselle Blackwell was shouted forth under the windows of my dormitory. You must know that these *sorties* are quite an event to the *élèves*; they gather about the happy departing one with all manner of good wishes for her enjoyment and safe return. So while one hooked my dress, another fastened my gloves, a third arranged my collar, the rest admired with the often repeated compliment, "Oh, que vous êtes belle!" and all sped me on my way with the pleasant greetings of their kind, light hearts.

How gay and free and delightful the city seemed to me after my four months' imprisonment—four months shut up within the high boundary wall of the institution, with the sky above the tops of tall houses only visible, and all life concentrated in a single subject! My chest seemed to grow broader as I stepped over the threshold and saw no barrier before me, but the beautiful Luxembourg Garden on one side, and unending streets on the other. The variety of busy life, the gay dresses, the cheerful houses, looked charming to me. I was surprised to find how strange everything seemed. I really saw Paris again for the first time, and criticised everything as on my first arrival. We walked down the long avenue that led from the observatory to the garden. On each side are nursery grounds on a much lower level than the great central avenue; they form a large lake of trees and flowers on each side the promenade. We descended into the beautiful flowery labyrinth to admire the magnificent dahlias of all colours and in immense quantities. The French are very fond of what they call *corbeilles*. There is one in every court of the Maternité; it is a large round plot of ground, filled to overflowing with every variety of bright flower, enclosed by a trellis-work that is covered inside and outside by morning glories, nasturtiums, &c., so that it is nothing but a hedge of flowers. The nursery grounds we walked through were full of these, which sent forth a delicious odour; and occasionally they were varied by an enclosed grass plot, hollowed out, and kept in the most beautiful order, with bright borders of flowers. As we ascended to the garden I was struck by the noble trees, dressed now in their varied autumn robes, through which the marble statues and antique palace sparkled as brightly as in the green summer time. We were saluted by showers of dead leaves, which gave the children much sport and the keepers much trouble. By the western gate is the immense block of buildings in which Anna has her pretty *appartement*. She introduced me to them, for the change of residence had been made since my retirement from the world, and I duly admired the elegant furniture, carved ceiling, tasteful paper, and above all the pretty look-out upon a long avenue of trees whose autumn foliage shed a warm glow through the rooms. At half-past twelve we hurried off to attend a magnetic *séance* at the Baron Dupotet's, which commenced precisely at one o'clock; and finding the omnibus too slow, we jumped into a cab with a lady who was bound on the same errand.

Now I must describe a magnetic *séance* to you; but I beg that you will receive the description with becoming seriousness, for I have a decided respect for M. Dupotet, and if any risibility should be excited it will proceed from your own nervous imagination, and not from my sober portraiture. These revelations of a higher sphere of existence are received up several pairs of stairs, in the back-room of a house situated in the heart of the city. It is a large, somewhat darkened room hung round with curious pictures, and lined with very curious people. Mesmer occupies a large frame carved with firebrands and anchors and other significant images; he looks fixedly at a pale lady hanging opposite to him, who has evidently undergone several magnetic crises. There are some verses framed and hanging very near the ceiling, surrounded by a thick wreath of yellow immortelles, but I have not yet been able to decipher their meaning. On the seats lining the walls about fifty persons assemble. It is an original assembly always, though it seems to be constantly changing. There was a lady with a small hole in her cheek, a child with a crooked neck, and the painter to the King of Sweden, with very light eyes and hair and great impressibility, with his companion who laughs and says, "Oui, monsieur," to every question addressed to him; and the son of the English Consul to Sicily, who displays a large amount of good clothes, good flesh, a little peaked moustache, and an immense amount of enthusiasm. But it would be difficult to give all the varieties of structure and expression in this group of believing heretics, some looking very fierce, some very sheepish, some with features turned up, some with them turned down, and some with them turned every way. The folding-doors of this room open into a small cabinet which is always opened on these occasions to receive Madame Dupotet and all the impressible ladies who form a circle inside, and go through many sympathetic manœuvres during the magnetising in the larger room: that is to say, the impressible ladies perform various antics, for Madame Dupotet, who is fat, fair, and forty, seems in no way affected, but looks on with smiling health and assists the nervous ladies. There was one remarkably fat dame, seated just within the folding-doors, who had powerful fits of nervous twitching, which gave her a singular appearance of pale, tremulous red jelly.

It would be impossible to describe the ornaments of M. Dupotet's study cabinet—the mystic symbols and black-letter books of the Black Art; but there is a little metallic mirror of oval form, traced with magic characters, which exerts a truly wonderful effect upon impressible subjects, exciting an ecstasy of delight or a transport of rage; but always an irresistible attraction for all who are affected by the magnetic influence. While M. Dupotet has been displaying it to the one particular object of his attention, half-a-dozen others steal up from all parts of the room to seize the prize; one little old lady under the magnetic influence came tottering up, with the drollest expression of violent jealousy on her face, and with her clenched fist prepared to fight the other equally eager disputants for the possession of this wonderful mirror.

Unfortunately, this particular meeting passed without any of those singular occurrences which are said sometimes to electrify the spectators. I heard much of the ecstasy of a young man which had thrilled every person present—believer or non-believer—the meeting before, in which the ordinary law of gravitation seemed to be superseded, and the entranced soul would actually have fled up into the heaven it was striving for had not M. Dupotet clasped the body tightly in his arms and commanded it back! But though no miracle was wrought, the faithful audience hung with intense interest on every manifestation of simple magnetic power; the aspiring features assumed a higher aspect, the downward ones bent more determinedly, and the red jelly became more tremulous at every fresh magnetisation; and when the *séance* closed everybody shook everybody's hand, and found it good to have been there.

Now, do not think my picture is a caricature—verily, I am very serious. There is an odd side to all reformers, to all who are pursuing a new idea earnestly, that is very whimsical. I am obliged to laugh at it; and yet I have true respect for M. Dupotet. Though he believes in ancient magic, though he lives in the hope of working miracles, I really believe him to be an honest, enthusiastic man, engaged with his whole soul in pursuing what seems to him the most important of all discoveries. His manner is perfectly unpretending, his conversation full of good sense; for twenty-five years he has pursued the same object, through suffering and ridicule and failure. He is honest, I am sure; how much truth he may possess I am at present quite unable to say; for my position, whilst it has given me occasional glimpses of his proceedings, has given no power of really investigating them; but some time I hope to really study magnetism.

As we walked back we stopped at the Louvre; I longed to see again that rich collection of art, particularly the statues, that seemed more beautiful than ever. We called in the Rue de Seine, hoping to gratify my old landlady, but she was out. Then Anna introduced me to her reading-room, where we studied the affairs of Europe, and grew indignant at the barbarism which seems for the moment triumphant. Anna took great pleasure all day in filling me with all manner of eatables, having great faith in "the very best beef," and I must confess that when dinner was concluded my dress felt a little tight at the waist!

Punctually at eight o'clock the recluse retired again from the vanities of the world. But, seriously, the idle day refreshed me; I needed it, and feel all the better for a little change.

October 24.—A most pleasant occurrence. Professor Lee, my Geneva Professor of Materia Medica, is in town, and is coming to see me to-morrow. He has been making a tour of two months in Great Britain, and now he visits Paris. How glad I shall be to see him, as a friend whom I respect, and with whom I can have a long delightful gossip! perhaps also he can give me information and some advice and introductions.

October 25.—By these most absurd regulations I was not allowed to show Dr. Lee over the hospital when he called. However, the *directeur* escorted him, and M. Blot offered an introduction to Ricord.

Although the residence in La Maternité was an extremely trying one from the utter absence of privacy, the poor air and food, and really hard work when sleep was lost on the average every fifth night, yet the medical experience was invaluable at that period of pioneer effort. It enabled me later to enter upon practice with a confidence in one important branch of medicine that no other period of study afforded; and I have always been glad that I entered the institution, notwithstanding the very grave accident which now befell me.

This event was noted at the time as follows:—

Sunday, November 4.—Served all day in the infirmary, and witnessed M. Dayau's first application of the serrefine. I felt all the afternoon a little grain of sand, as it were, in one eye. I was afraid to think what it might be, for in the dark early morning, whilst syringing the eye of one of my tiny patients for purulent ophthalmia, some of the water had spurted into my own eye. It was much swollen at night, and in the morning the lids were closely adherent from suppuration.

November 5.—I applied for permission to leave until the eye was well, and was refused. I went to the infirmary of the *élèves* and informed M. Blot that I was prisoner. He examined the eye carefully, discovered that it was the dreaded disease, consulted his chief, and then told me that as everything depended on the early active treatment, he should give up the first days entirely to me. He expressed much sympathy, arranged everything for me in the most thoughtful way, and I went to bed—I little knew for how long! I despatched a note to my sister, and then active treatment commenced—the eyelids cauterised, leeches to the temple, cold compresses, ointment of belladonna, opium to the forehead, purgatives, footbaths, and sinapisms, with broth for diet. The eye was syringed every hour, and I realised the danger of the disease from the weapons employed against it. Poor Anna came down in the evening to sympathise with the "inflamed eye" I had written about, and was dreadfully shocked. She has told me since how many times she hid behind the curtain to cry. My friendly young doctor came every two hours, day and night, to tend the eye, Mlle. Mallet acting in the alternate hours. The infirmary was kept profoundly quiet, and a guard appointed day and night. The sympathy was universal and deep, the *élèves* asking after me with tears. An unheard-of permission was granted to Anna to visit me three times a day. For three days this continued—then the disease had done its worst; and I learned from the tone of my friends that my eye was despaired of. Ah! how dreadful it was to find the daylight gradually fading as my kind doctor bent over me, and removed with an exquisite delicacy of touch the films that had formed over the pupil! I could see him for a moment clearly, but the sight soon vanished, and the eye was left in darkness.

For three weeks I lay in bed with both eyes closed, then the right eye began to open gradually, and I could get up and do little things for myself. How kind everybody was! I shall never forget it. Anna, with her faith in magnetism, came down regularly three times a day in rain and snow to sympathise and impart "the vital fluid." My friendship deepened for my young physician, and I planned a little present for his office. Madame Charrier entered into it with spirit; we had long discussions together, and finally secured an elegant pair of lamps for his consultation-rooms, which I hurried through the corridors to see, bundled up in my dressing-gown and shawl, looking and feeling very much like a ghost. The lamps were conveyed to his room that night. The next morning he came to me evidently full of delight, and longing to be amiable, yet too conscientious to infringe the rules of the Maternité by acknowledging the present. He admired my braid of long hair, wondered how fingers without eyes could arrange anything so beautifully regular; spoke of the Protestant religion, thought if he joined any Church it would be that; turned to go, turned back again, and was evidently hardly able to leave without thanking me. Mlle. Mallet told me that the night before he had run in to Madame Charrier to tell her of his present, and on his way out passed by the cloisters in an evident perplexity, longing to enter the infirmary of the *élèves*, but unable to do so. I do admire his delicate conscientiousness!

I received a visit from M. Davenne, who had sent me a message of sympathy. I could not clearly make him out with my dim eye, but had a general idea of a short, elderly man standing hat in hand, and regarding me as one would a solemn religious spectacle. M. Boivin made some very friendly remarks to me, and concluded, raising his hand, "et, voyez-vous? c'est d'une patience."

"Angélique!" replied M. Davenne.

Saturday, 22nd.—Oh, how happy I am at this moment, for Dubois has just left me, understanding for the first time the justice of my determination to obtain a full medical education, and obliged to confess that I was right in principle. I shall have my *congé*, and a hope of *cliniques* and study in the Eccentric hospitals. Heaven has answered that heart-cry of the other night.

Wednesday, 26th.—Off actually! I dressed for the first time. Bandaged and veiled; the carriage drove to the door, Anna guided me in. I made kind adieus, caught glimpses of stone walls in the cold dull light, and thus ended my Maternité life. I felt very weak, and laughed hysterically the whole evening.

The following letter, written at this time to an uncle, an officer in the British army, shows the important support which the mind can render the body in combating disease:—

DEAR UNCLE,—I thank you with all my heart for the kind sympathy you have expressed for me so warmly. Fate certainly gave me a strange and sudden blow, but now I am up again strong and hopeful, and eager for work, I beg uncle to feel quite sure that a brave soldier's niece will never disgrace the colours she fights under; but will be proud of the wounds gained in a great cause, and resolve more strongly than ever to "conquer or die." In truth, dear friends, the accident might have been so much worse that I am more disposed to rejoice than to complain. Even in its present state the eye is not a very striking disfigurement, and it will gradually become still less so. As to the more serious consideration—loss of vision—I still hope to recover that in time, and meanwhile the right eye grows daily stronger. I can write without difficulty, read a little, and hope soon to resume my usual employments. I certainly esteem myself very fortunate, and I still mean to be at no very distant day *the first lady surgeon in the world.*

I find from your letters that there is a possibility of your visiting Paris. I should rejoice in the prospect of meeting you, if my own stay were certain; but it is by no means so. I have already accomplished much in France, but I find it very difficult to proceed further; still, I cannot yet judge decidedly of my prospects. I have just received permission from Government to visit the hospitals, which is encouraging, and one opening may lead to others, so that I may still hope to meet you some day, unless you should grow frightened at the idea of my scalpel and lancet, and feel uncertain how far the ties of relationship may modify the experimental researches of the medical student!

Believe me, very truly,

Your niece,

ELIZABETH BLACKWELL.

But the six months which followed my departure from the Maternité proved to be a time of great mental suffering, under which a strong physical constitution threatened to give way; for the condition of the affected organ entirely prevented that close application to professional study which was needed. Both anatomical and surgical work were out of the question; and even reading had to be laid aside. I followed a few lectures and some *cliniques* at the Hôtel-Dieu, by permission of M. Roux, and engaged a *répétiteur*, but this was quite inadequate to accomplish the end in view.

In June of 1850 a visit to the fine mountain air of Priessnitz's famous establishment at Gräfenberg was resolved on, in the hope of regaining strength and power of study. Travelling rapidly through France, Germany, and Prussia, in five days I reached the famous water-cure region. On the journey a day had been spent in Berlin, where I had been struck by the arrogance of the Prussian officers, and the fear which was expressed by a friend with whom I talked freely in Kroll's Garden lest conversation should be overheard!

Freiwaldau, at the foot of the Gräfenberg, was full of

Kurgäste; but, being warned by a lady to whom I brought an introduction that it would be impossible for a lady to go alone to the Gräfenberg Hotel, for it "was full of gentlemen who went about in their shirt-sleeves," I was rather perplexed as to where to go. A home letter describes this curious experience:—

Gräfenberg, 3 P.M.—On a shady seat on the brow of a hill commanding a most beautiful prospect. Dearly beloved people, this cometh to you from a very watery person in a very watery place. The sound of water is heard everywhere. But I must give you some particulars. Not being able to find lodgings in Freiwaldau, I left word for Priessnitz to call, and was sitting in my little upper room at the hotel, feeling decidedly blue, when the door opened and in walked a middle-sized, elderly man, with sun-burnt face marked with the smallpox, with grey hair, light-blue eyes, a pleasant expression of face, and dressed in country-best style. I liked his appearance, 'twas honest and good. He examined me very closely with his little blue eyes all the time I was explaining my wishes. Then, in his abrupt manner, he told me he could make me quite strong in about six weeks, and the cure would do no harm to my eye. When I told him that I was informed Gräfenberg was quite full, he said, "You *can* come, child; come this afternoon, and bring your things with you," and off he went. I felt quite relieved to be spared the bother of lodging-hunting and housekeeping. I determined to face the innumerable gentlemen in shirt sleeves, and let properness go; if the *Gräfinn* did not like my position—why, she might dislike it! When I reached the place of my destination I was a little confounded. At the very top of the house, with bare rafters for the roof and the wall, a row of little windows a foot high let into the roof above my head, a wooden crib full of straw, three wooden chairs, a table, and low bureau with a green earthenware bowl; this was my room and its furniture. I must have looked rather dismayed, for the girl hastened to inform me that I had an Italian count and countess for my next-door neighbours, and that there were eight ladies and eight gentlemen on the same floor, and that we should be out in the woods all day. Of course I could say nothing when I found I had such noble neighbours, or rather when I found that it was really the last vacant room in the house!

When the bell rang for tea I was shown into an immense hall that might seat 500 people, gaily painted, and ornamented with chandeliers. I sat down and found myself, to my utter amazement, beside a row of ladies in grand toilette gossamer dresses with short sleeves and waists a *little lower* than I thought waists were ever worn; hair dressed out with curls and flowers, bracelets (I counted five on the arm next me) and rings to match! The long tables were covered with alternate bowls of sour and sweet milk, and brown bread and butter. The bread looked inviting, but when, with difficulty, I had sawn off a morsel, it was so sour that I could hardly swallow it; but the milk was good, and I did it justice. People kept coming in in groups, very merry, but all talking German; the gentlemen, I presume, were in shirt sleeves, but as they were all covered with coats, I was not shocked!

The next morning early I went through a series of hydropathic operations, at which Priessnitz assisted, as he always does the first time. The course never varied—viz. packing, a half-bath, a plunge bath, a wet bandage, and some glasses of cold water at six o'clock; an *Abreibung*, sitz bath, and another wet bandage at twelve o'clock; ditto at four P.M., and water *ad libitum* all through the day.

The diet is plain, but every morning an old woman opens a white-bread shop outside the dining-room, to which almost every one is customer. Each one comes in from the early morning walk, buys a roll, and marches in with it under his arm; and morning and evening the little strawberry gatherers offer the Alpine strawberries, with their fine wild-wood flavour, for sale.

Everybody seems to have a good appetite. My own is ravenous; a half-day in the open air, rambling over these fine mountain-sides, stimulated by the wind and the abundant really living water, I find myself suddenly in strong, vigorous health, and the idea of sickness seems a fable.

At first I felt very lonely in such a large assembly; but now I speak to a good many, and I have found one young American, Mr. Glynn, who seems like a brother in this concourse of strangers. He is about twenty-two, nearly blind from amaurosis, but one of the "smartest" fellows I have ever met; quick as a flash, full of Yankee shrewdness, he bears his terrible misfortune with real heroism, and has rendered me numberless little services.

There are several mountain-sides laid out with walks innumerable. The favourite early morning walk is to the Priessnitz spring; you wind round and up the mountain, partly through open, sweet-smelling fields, partly through pleasant fir woods, passing several springs by the way, each with its name and inscription and rustic seats around; at each you stop and drink, chat a little with those you meet, and perhaps sit down for a few moments. It is very sweet at this hour: the leaves smell so fresh, the beautiful flowers are covered with dew, and the cuckoo is heard in the woods all day. This stroll generally occupies two hours. . . .

It is very amusing to watch the people. Gräfenberg is the rage in Germany; all classes are represented here. The Countess von Westhalp offers to introduce me to a fashionable English circle in Freiwaldau, headed by Lady Darley; and to our great indignation the "butcher" Haynau, notorious for his barbarities, made his appearance here one day. In the house we have gymnasium, billiard-room, library, theatre, and balls frequently take place. . . .

Priessnitz has 500 patients under his care, and with their friends they amount to hundreds more. You see him sitting at the head of one of the large tables, three times a day, looking very pleasant. He is quiet and simple in manner, but has a very determined mouth. They say he is proud of having been an Austrian serf. His pleasant-looking daughter is married to an Hungarian baron.

These foreign titles are really a farce. I am here in my loft one day, in slippers and old dressing-gown, when a knock comes to my door. When I open it, a tall, black-whiskered foreigner appears, who presents the respects of Mme. la Princesse Obolenska, and hopes I will call upon her when I next go to Freiwaldau. The man made quite sure that I was I—as well he might, for I never had quite such queer surroundings. . . . I paid my visit, a professional one, after all. I had to put up with four gulden, instead of the honour; but she was a simple, pleasant lady, and we parted on the pleasantest terms. This was, in fact, my first regular professional consultation.

The air and water, however, of that lovely region, with the constant outdoor life and endless rambles over the Bohemian mountain-sides, proved too stimulating to the still sensitive organ: a violent attack of inflammation supervened. With great difficulty I returned to Paris, and placed myself under the care of the famous oculist Desmarres. This gentleman rendered me the most skilful and generous aid. In the course of a few weeks he restored me to active work again, although the sight of one eye was permanently lost, and the intention of making surgery a speciality necessarily abandoned.

During this trying period of Parisian study, my cousin, Mr. Kenyon Blackwell, a South Staffordshire ironmaster, was endeavouring to promote my strong desire to study in one of our London hospitals. He applied to the able and highly esteemed dean of St. Bartholomew's Hospital, who presented the application to the treasurer. The subject was referred to the Medical Council of the hospital. The result was forwarded to me as follows:—

At a House Committee held on Tuesday, the 14th day of May, 1850, a letter addressed to the treasurer from Mr. Paget, communicating to him the request of Miss Elizabeth Blackwell, a lady well connected in this country and the United States, to attend as a student in the wards and other departments of the hospital, was read, when the treasurer reported that the same had been referred to the Medical Council, and the opinion of all the members of the council having been read, and Mr. Paget having attended and furnished the committee with such information as was required, it was resolved:

"That in the opinion of this committee Miss Blackwell should be admitted as a student under such regulations as the treasurer and almoners may from time to time deem necessary."

James Paget, Esq.

The ticket of admission forwarded at the same time granted permission to study in any ward, and follow the visit of any physician or surgeon who was willing to extend to me the facilities of his department. The permission was accompanied by a cordial welcome from the dean, Mr. James Paget, M.R.C.S.

This was indeed joyful news. I could now in an open and honourable way, no longer regarded with suspicion, but protected by the highest medical sanction, devote myself to the unlimited field of practical medicine so cordially thrown open to me, and which I ardently desired to study. I hastened to London, and, after some little difficulty in obtaining lodgings, on account of being a lady, alone, established myself in rooms in Thavies Inn, then a delightfully quiet set of houses, entered by an archway from busy Holborn.

Every morning after breakfast I now regularly betook myself to the hospital, spending many hours there daily, and making the Faith wards, under Dr. Burrows, my headquarters; but Messrs. Lawrence, Stanley, and Lloyd courteously welcomed me to their wards. Indeed, every department was cordially opened to me, *except the department for female diseases!*

Kind old Dr. Hue was always ready to show me cases of interest, and he took me by an underground passage, which led to Christ's Hospital, to taste the famous pea-soup made for the lads of that old Foundation school.

I particularly valued the special visits of clinical observation, without students, which Dr. Baly and Mr. Kirkes were making.

Mr. Kirkes was preparing a new edition of his excellent "Student's Physiology," and Dr. Baly was pursuing his valuable investigations on dysentery. In relation to the latter, it is noted in my journal: "He is so gentle, so friendly, and so learned in his art, that he teaches me more than anyone else."

I also attended Mr. Paget's admirable lectures on pathological anatomy, given in the amphitheatre. My seat there was always courteously reserved for me. I experienced also the utmost consideration from the students, a large class of whom always followed Dr. Burrows's visits. Indeed, so natural did this innovation of a lady student soon become, that when, the following year, I paid my farewell visit to the treasurer, he remarked, to my great gratification, "Why, we had quite forgotten you were here!"

Many home letters mark the various incidents of this extremely interesting period of study.

London, 28 Thavies Inn: November 1.

DEAR FRIENDS,—When I arrived in London on October 3, I was actually dismayed by the intolerable atmosphere, the dense envelope of foggy smoke that made me sick during the day and kept me awake at night; and as I continued to make observations on persons and things, and finally settled down in my present prosaic lodgings, I asked myself with astonishment, Is this the same London I saw a year and a half ago, or is it a different person examining the same objects? But now, happily, that state of forlornity has passed away. I have almost forgotten the smoke; my lodgings are clean and convenient. I am making friends, and I shall use all the opportunities I can get for studying social subjects and seeing society, provided they do not interfere with my work and are not too expensive.

My first introduction to St. Bartholomew's was at a breakfast at Mr. Paget's. He has a house within the hospital boundaries, and a special oversight of the students. At the commencement of each session he invites the students to breakfast in parties of about a dozen, and to one of those breakfasts I, on my arrival, was invited. The students seemed to be gentlemanly fellows, and looked with some curiosity at their new companion; the conversation was general and pleasant, the table well covered, Mrs. Paget very sensible and agreeable, so that it was quite a satisfactory time. Soon after I was invited to meet a distinguished German gentleman, Professor Kölliker, whom I found most agreeable and intelligent. My old acquaintance, Professor Owen, entertained us with traditions of London. Dr. Carpenter was also present, and some of the older students, looking very amiable, though awkward. The gentlemen I find more friendly than the ladies; I fear I shall find them in the shocked phase this winter. There are, however, a few decided exceptions. . . .

But now I am going to tell mother of a visit which I made yesterday on purpose to amuse her—viz. to our old Bridge Street minister, Dr. Leifchild, whose christening of me I distinctly remember! Between three and four, on my return from hospital, I set out determined to hunt up the family, and after searching directories and trudging several miles, and being wrongly directed, when I finally inquired at No. 5 Camden Street, a quiet, respectable house, whether Dr. Leifchild was in, I listened with great relief to the announcement that he was probably taking his nap. I was ushered into a large plainly furnished parlour, where sat Mrs. Leifchild, sewing by a round table in the middle. My childish recollection had retained a general impression of the person, though I should not have recognised her. She is seventy-two, and wearing spectacles, but does not look more than fifty, so fresh, plump, and pretty, though unfortunately so deaf that she could only hear an occasional word. I announced myself. She replied, "I remember the family well. Mr. Blackwell was deacon in the chapel. You are one of his sisters." I could hardly make her believe that I was third *daughter*. She remembered A. and M. well; said they were clever girls; she knew they would turn out something remarkable, but she had no recollection of me. Their son John came in at that moment—a tall, thin man, reminding me of the Lane Seminary student, Jones. I don't know whether I ever saw him before. Of course the doctor was sent for to see the stranger. I recognised him at once, and should have known him anywhere—fat, rosy, and laughing, notwithstanding his grey hair. I did not detect anything of the old man in him. "Ah," said he, "I know that face," and then he made me take my bonnet off and occupy a large chair by the fire, and tell him all about the family, and particularly my mother. "A sweet creature she was! How I should like to see her again! Doesn't she talk about visiting England? I wish she would." He spoke of father with great affection, as a true friend. He had received most beautiful letters from him. "If my memoirs are published, one of his letters will appear in them." They had been told that the two eldest Miss Blackwells were very dashing girls, and wanted to know the truth. Then, why had I come to England? I told him I had been doing a rather singular thing; I had been studying medicine. He looked at me to see if I were in earnest, and then burst out into such a hearty, merry laugh that I joined in with all my might. "Yes, I had obtained a diploma as doctor in medicine." "You—doctor!" and then another hearty laugh. Of course Mrs. Leifchild wanted to know what we were laughing at. "Why, my dear, that girl there is Doctor in Medicine!" and then I must give them the whole history; and I certainly never had three more attentive listeners, interrupted by the doctor's exclamations: "Bless me, what she has done; what she has suffered! Why, the girl's a genius! Where did she get it all from? Why, no man could have done what she has done!" And if ever I stopped, John would say, "Now, Miss Blackwell, pray go on; it's the most interesting narrative I ever listened to; you left off at Paris." I was much amused. To that little family, who had been staying so quietly at home in the same routine, it did sound like a romance. When I had done, the doctor declared "it was a capital thing—it was the beginning of a new era." And John at once brought out pen and paper and begged me to give him my autograph. The doctor said the Rev. Mr. May, from America, was an old friend and class-mate who had visited England about two years ago, and he graphically described their interview. When Dr. L. opened the door, he started back. "No! Yes! It isn't—it is! It can't be possible! It is very certain; but won't you let me in?" From Mr. May he learned that the eldest of the Blackwells had become Socinians; and then I must give an account of my religious faith. Of course I spoke up for myself. I told him my religion was certainly a little peculiar; but nevertheless it was a very good and very strong one—and he didn't seem much troubled about the state of my soul; indeed, I believe that, on the whole, he considered that it was a little safer than most of the ladies' of his acquaintance! So, mother, I beg you to take the same view of the matter. Altogether, I met with the heartiest reception. The doctor placed all his influence at my service, and Mrs. Leifchild will write you all the news of your old Bristol friends. So I hope you approve of my calling. . . .

Now I am writing in a queer place—viz. one of the wards of St. Bartholomew's, whilst awaiting the visit of one of the physicians. This famous old hospital is only five minutes' walk from my lodgings, and every morning, as the clock strikes nine, I walk down Holborn Hill, make a short cut through the once famous Cock Lane, and find myself at a gate of the hospital that enables me to enter with only a side glance at Smithfield Cattle Market. "Punch" had really frightened me by his account of the dangerous tumult of animals; but, happily, I need only glance across the open space, forgetting the bulls, pigs, &c., that occupy it now, and also the fearful fires of persecution once lighted there, and try to bring back the time when it was lined with gay tents, and surrounded by galleries filled with beauty, eager to witness the brilliant encounters of arms that took place there in the age of tournaments. Now a little dark figure with doctorial sack and writing-case under arm makes its way through assembling students, who politely step aside to let it pass, and entering the museum, studies its numerous preparations till the hour of lecture, when an attendant shows it to a seat. I only attend regularly one course of lectures—viz. Mr. Paget's very interesting course on pathology. Mr. Paget spoke to the students before I joined the class. When I entered and bowed, I received a round of applause. My seat is always reserved for me, and I have no trouble. There are, I think, about sixty students, the most gentlemanly class I have ever seen. I have been here about ten days. There are so many physicians and surgeons, so many wards, and all so exceedingly busy, that I have not yet got the run of the place; but the medical wards are thrown open unreservedly to me, either to follow the physician's visits or for private study; later, I shall attend the surgical wards. At first no one knew how to regard me. Some thought I must be an extraordinary intellect overflowing with knowledge; others, a queer, eccentric woman; and none seemed to understand that I was a quiet, sensible person who had acquired a small amount of medical knowledge, and who wished by patient observation and study acquire considerably more. One of the old physicians takes much interest in the strange little doctor, and has given me valuable hints from his own experience; but I confess that this system of practice is both difficult and repellent to me; I shall, however, study it diligently. Mr. Paget, who is very cordial, tells me that I shall have to encounter much more prejudice from ladies than from gentlemen in my course. I am prepared for this. Prejudice is more violent the blinder it is, and I think that Englishwomen seem wonderfully shut up in their habitual views. But a work of the ages cannot be hindered by individual feeling. A hundred years hence women will not be what they are now.

The growing perplexity of the conscientious student awakening to the uncertainty of the art of medicine is now apparent in letters written at this time.

November 20, 1850.

DEAR E.,—I want to talk to you seriously about the future—that is to say, my *medical future*. It has been a heavy, perplexing subject to me on what system I should practise, for the old one appeared to me wrong, and I have even thought every heresy better; but since I have been looking into these heresies a little more closely I feel as dissatisfied with them as with the old one. We hear of such wonderful cures continually being wrought by this and the other thing, that we forget on how small a number the novelty has been exercised, and the failures are never mentioned; but on the same principle, I am convinced that if the old system were the heresy, and the heresy the established custom, we should hear the same wonders related of the drugs. Neither hydropathy nor mesmerism are what their enthusiastic votaries imagine them to be. At Gräfenberg I could not hear of one case of perfect cure, and unfortunately the undoubtedly great resources of cold water are not so developed and classified as to enable a young practitioner to introduce it, professedly, into his practice. Mesmerism has not converted me since watching its effects on patients. I do wish most heartily that I could discover more of the remedial agency of magnetism, for my conviction is that it ought to be powerfully beneficial in some cases; and as I find they have a magnetic dispensary here in London, I shall certainly try and attend it frequently. I am sorry that I have been unable hitherto to attend more to homœpathy, the third heresy of the present time, but I am trying now to find out opportunities. Here I have been following now with earnest attention, for a few weeks, the practice of a very large London hospital, and I find the majority of patients do get well; so I have come to this conclusion—that I must begin with a practice which is an old-established custom, which has really more expressed science than any other system; but nevertheless, as it dissatisfies me heartily, I shall commence as soon as possible building up a hospital in which I can experiment; and the very instant I feel *sure* of any improvement I shall adopt it in my practice, in spite of a whole legion of opponents. Now E., future partner, what say you—is it not the only rational course? If I were rich I would not begin private practice, but would only experiment; as, however, I am poor, I have no choice. I look forward with great interest to the time when you can aid me in these matters, for I have really no *medical friend*; all the gentlemen I meet seem separated by an invincible barrier, and women who take up the subject partially are inferior. It will not always be so; when the novelty of the innovation is past, men and women will be valuable friends in medicine, but for a time that cannot be. I spend now about three or four hours each day in the wards, chiefly medical, diagnosing disease, watching the progress of cases, and accustoming my ear to the stethoscope. Already, in this short time, I feel that I have made progress, and detect sounds that I could not distinguish on my entrance. I advise you, E., to familiarise yourself with the healthy sounds of the chest. When you go home, auscultate all the family; you will find quite a variety in the sounds, though all may be healthy persons. Lay a cloth over the chest and listen with the ear simply; it is as good as a stethoscope with clean people. I wish I could lend you my little black stethoscope that I brought from the Maternité.

I have been disappointed in one thing here—the Professor of Midwifery and the Diseases of Women and Children wrote me a very polite note, telling me that he entirely disapproved of a lady's studying medicine, and begging me to consider that his neglecting to give me aid was owing to no disrespect to me as a lady, but to his condemnation of my object.

By-the-by, I must tell you of a scientific explanation of the toughness of meat which I obtained from Mr. Paget's lecture the other morning; it arises from cooking meat during the *rigor mortis*! Would not that be a delicate suggestion for a squeamish individual? . . .

28 Thavies Inn: 1850.

Dear Dr. Dickson,—I believe that my kind preceptor and earliest medical friend will be interested in a little account of my foreign life.

My request for permission to attend St. Bartholomew's Hospital was cordially granted, and I have received a friendly welcome from professors and students. I have the full rights of a student granted to me. I do not attend many of the lectures, but confine my attention chiefly to the practice of the hospital, and at present, more particularly, to the medical practice. If I remain through the summer, I shall gradually extend my visits to the surgical and other wards, as I am particularly anxious to become widely acquainted with disease. I am obliged to feel very sceptical as to the wisdom of much of the practice which I see pursued every day. I try very hard to believe, I continually call up my own inexperience and the superior ability of the physicians whose actions I am watching; but my doubts will not be subdued, and render me the more desirous of obtaining the bedside knowledge of sickness which will enable me to *commit heresy* with intelligence in the future, if my convictions impel me to it. I hope you will forgive this confession of want of faith, which I do not venture to make to my present instructors, for the English are in general too conservative to have sympathy with unbelief, however honest.

I do not find so active a spirit of investigation in the English professors as in the French. In Paris this spirit pervaded young and old, and gave a wonderful fascination to the study of medicine, which even

I, standing only on the threshold, strongly felt. There are innumerable medical societies there, and some of the members are always *on the eve* of most important discoveries; a brilliant theory is *almost* proved, and creates intense interest; some new plan of treatment is always exciting attention in the hospitals, and its discussion is widely spread by the immense crowds of students freely admitted. The noble provision of free lectures, supported by the French Government, increases this tendency; the distinguished men who fill the chairs in these institutions have all the leisure and opportunity necessary for original investigation, and a receptive audience always ready to reflect the enthusiasm of the teacher. I have often listened to some of these eloquent men in the College of France, their natural eloquence increased by the novelty or brilliant suggestions of the subject, till I shared fully in the enthusiasm of the assembly; and then, in the excited feeling of the moment, I would enter with some friend into the beautiful adjacent garden of the Luxembourg, and, sitting down at the foot of some noble statue, we would prolong the interest by discussion; while the brilliant atmosphere, the trees, the wind and the water, the fine old palace and the varied groups of people moving amongst the flowers, contributed to the charm of the moment, producing some of the intensest pleasurable sensations I have ever enjoyed. I cannot wonder that students throng to Paris, instead of to the immense smoke-hidden London; here there is no excitement, all moves steadily onward, constantly but without enthusiasm. No theory sets the world on fire till it is well established, and the German observers are much more studied than the French. Everything is stamped by good sense and clear substantial thought; my respect is fully commanded, but I often long for a visit to the College of France and a stroll in the Luxembourg.

Whilst devoting all my daytime to the rare advantage of practical study so providentially opened to me, the evenings were in another direction equally delightful and beneficial. I was sitting, one dull afternoon, in my bare lodging-house drawing-room, somewhat regretfully thinking of the bright skies of Paris and pleasant study under the trees of the Luxembourg Garden, when the door opened and three young ladies entered, and introduced themselves as Miss Bessie Rayner Parkes and the Misses Leigh Smith.

This proved the commencement of a lifelong friendship. These ladies were filled with a noble enthusiasm for the responsible and practical work of women in the various duties of life. They warmly sympathised in my medical effort, and were connected with that delightful society of which Lady Noel Byron, Mrs. Follen, Mrs. Jameson, the Herschels, and Faraday were distinguised members, and with which the Rev. Mr. Morris and the Hon. Russell Gurney were in full sympathy.

My young friends hung my dull rooms with their charming paintings, made them gay with flowers, and welcomed me to their family circles with the heartiest hospitality.

A bright social sun henceforth cheered the somewhat sombre atmosphere of my hospital life; for when the day's duties were accomplished there was always some pleasant social gathering, or some concert or lecture attended with friends, to refresh the medical student. I often walked home from my friends in the West between twelve and one at night (being too poor to engage cabs), not exhausted, but invigorated for the next day's work. Lady Noel Byron became warmly interested in my studies. I went with her to Faraday's lectures, visited her at Brighton, and she long remained one of my correspondents.

One of my most valued acquaintances was Miss Florence Nightingale, then a young lady at home, but chafing against the restrictions that crippled her active energies. Many an hour we spent by my fireside in Thavies Inn, or walking in the beautiful grounds of Embley, discussing the problem of the present and hopes of the future. To her, chiefly, I owed the awakening to the fact that sanitation is the supreme goal of medicine, its foundation and its crown.

My acquaintance also with Professor Georgii, the Swedish professor of kinesipathy and the favourite disciple of Brandt, whose consultation-rooms in Piccadilly I often visited, strengthened my faith in the employment of hygienic measures in medicine. When, in later years, I entered into practice, extremely sceptical in relation to the value of drugs and ordinary medical methods, my strong faith in hygiene formed the solid ground from which I gradually built up my own methods of treatment. Looking back upon a long medical life, one of my happiest recollections is of the number of mothers whom I influenced in the healthy education of their children.

Letters written home at this date indicate the vivid interests of the time.

November 1850.

DEAR E.,—The great topics of the day here are the Great Industrial Exhibition and Popery.

On November 5 the bells were ringing and the boys hurrahing for "Gunpowder Plot Day." This anniversary was celebrated with more enthusiasm than usual from the Pope's having appointed a Cardinal Archbishop of England, and "No Popery" placards are posted everywhere.

The great building of iron and glass for the Exhibition is rapidly rising in Hyde Park, and the papers in this rank-loving country duly inform us whenever Prince Albert comes in from Windsor to inspect its progress, and furthermore that the Prince is modelling a group of statuary, and the Queen designing a carpet, to figure in the display. The last time I was at the Twamleys' we drove round to see the building, which is a curious sight from the delicate appearance of the immense quantity of iron framework; it looks too fragile to support a crowd, and yet it will hold myriads. There is a splendid old elm tree which they have enclosed in the building, and his great black arms look in strange contrast to the surrounding tracery.

December 24, 1850.

DEAR M.,—I was just stretching myself after breakfast, and thinking that I must put on my boots and turn out into the horrible fog that was darkening daylight, when your welcome letters came, and it being holiday time I treated myself to an immediate perusal. I must beg you not to imagine me sitting in a large bare room in an *inn*. The term "inn" is only applied in this case to a particularly quiet and respectable little street. The term "Inns of Court" means a number of buildings round an open court, withdrawn from the street, entered by an arched passage under some house, and used now or at some former time for law purposes. That was the origin of Thavies Inn; it was formerly a portion of an old law court, and is particularly *proper*, having iron gates at the archway, which are shut at night, and a porter living in the little house at the entrance, who is always on the look-out for beggars or other un-respectable characters; and the way in which a little barrel organ that has managed to slip in is "shut up." at the first bar has always amused me, and provoked me at the same time. The room also, which was bare enough at first, has assumed a much more homelike aspect since two young friends sent me some pictures to hang on the walls, and a portfolio of paintings, with a little stand on which to place a new one every day; and having turned the sideboard into a bookcase, I can assure you it looks quite comfortable when I have drawn the round table to the fire and settled down for the evening.

Your letter alludes to many topics of interest. First of all this "Woman's Rights Convention," held at Worcester, Mass. I have read through all the proceedings carefully. They show great energy, much right feeling, but not, to my judgement, a great amount of strong, clear thought. This last, of course, one ought not to expect in the beginning; but in my own mind I have settled it as a society to respect, to feel sympathy for, to help incidentally, but not—for me—to work with body and soul. I cannot sympathise fully with an anti-man movement. I have had too much kindness, aid, and just recognition from men to make such attitude of women otherwise than painful; and I think the true end of freedom may be gained better in another way. I was touched by the kind rememberance of W.H.C., which placed my name on the Industrial Committee; and if I were in America and called on to attend I should certainly send them a note full of respect and sympathy; but I must keep my energy for what seems to me a deeper movement. But I think you did perfectly right to act on the Education Committee, and if I can send you any information I will gladly do so. But I feel a little perplexed by the main object of the Convention—Woman's Rights. The great object of education has nothing to do with woman's rights, or man's rights, but with the development of the human soul and body. But let me know how you mean to treat the subject, and I will render you what aid I can. . . . My head is full of the idea of organisation, but not organisation of women in opposition to men. I have been lately meditating constantly on this idea, and seeking some principle of organisation which should be a constantly growing one, until it became adequate to meet the wants of the time. . . . This horrible fact of immorality has weighed upon fearfully since I came to London, for I believe in no city in the world does it show itself so *publicly* as it does here. In Paris it is legalised and hidden, and is recognised and profitable as a branch of the Government!

In the United States it is not so old and widespread (written in 1850); but here in London it has been let alone, has taken an unrestrained course, exists to a fearful extent, and shows itself conspiciously in its lowest form. At all hours of the night I see groups of our poor wretched sisters, standing at every corner of the streets, decked out in their best, which best is generally a faded shawl and even tattered dress, seeking their wretched living; and many aching hearts I have seen looking through the thin, hungry features. But I will not pain you farther; you know the general fact, though you have never had it pressed home to you in a thousand ways, as I have. My great dream is of a grand moral reform society, a wide movement of women in this matter; the remedy to be sought in every sphere of life—radical action—not the foolish application of plasters, that has hitherto been the work of the so-called "moral reform" societies; we must leave the present castaway, but redeem the rising generation. In my own mind I have divided my "Union" into many branches, several of which I see Mr. Channing has proposed for this "Woman's Rights Society." Education to change both the male and female perverted character; industrial occupation, including formation of a priesthood of women; colonial operations, clubs, homes, social unions, a true Press, and many other things, have been among my visions; and the whole so combined that it could be brought to bear on any outrage or prominent evil. In England I should seek to interest the Queen, and place her, as the highest representative of womanhood, at the head of this grand moral army. Indeed, many of my modifications naturally fit themselves to English society, which is immediately around one. When I return to America, of course the European mould of my thoughts will drop off, and fit itself to the New World; but it never can be an anti-man movement. . . . One thing now pleases me much; all the women seem to like me, from the aristocratic Miss Montgomery, bosom friend of one of the Queen's maids of honour, down to the humble sisters of the hospital, all welcome me, and many with enthusiasm. I have passed several delightful evenings with Mrs. Follen, Mrs. Jameson, and the Chapmans; the De Morgans, Morells, and many others are unceasing in their kindness. I find these people varying in religion and everything else, but all alive and open to progressive ideas—if they are not shocked back. There seems to be a very large class of this kind, who are not united in any special effort, but in whom the true ideas are germinating, which will some time—perhaps in their children, for things move slowly in England—reach a perfect development. It is my *impression*, for I ought only to put it in that modest form, that the corresponding class in America is less humane, more addicted to money-getting and party spirit; and that reform ideas in America are much more talked of, but less acted on. . . .

April 4, 1851.

Dear E.,—I have been very gay lately, with so many social entertainments. One evening at the Hon. Miss Murray's I saw the Duchess of Buckingham, Duke of Argyll, Marquis of Lansdowne, and many distinguished people, Sir Lyon Playfair, Sir John Herschel, the Speaker of the House of Commons, &c. But my studies go steadily on, and I do enjoy going round with Dr. Baly; he is so gentle and friendly, and so learned in his art, that he teaches me more than anyone else. I wish I could go round with him oftener. . . .

But I must tell you of a delightful three days' visit that I made to Lady Byron at Brighton a week ago. I had heard her most highly spoken of, and her connection with the poet has thrown a romance around her; so when I received through Miss Montgomery an invitation from her, stating that she had herself paid some attention to medical matters and would be most happy to see me, and that her friend Dr. King would do the honours of the well-arranged hospital at Brighton, I determined to accept, and give myself a three days' treat. I arrived in Brighton one bright, blowing afternoon. Nearly three miles of good stone houses face the broad sea, the road in front of them forming a delightful elevated promenade open to the spray and the Atlantic winds. In the distance at one extremity was Beachy Head, at the other the projecting point that hid Portsmouth, and far out, dim in the distance, lay the Isle of Wight. Bare, rounded, green hills formed the background to the town. In the bow-windowed parlour of one of these large stone houses I was set down, and soon after, Lady Byron, who had been to the railroad to look for me, entered—a slender, rather small, but venerable-looking lady of sixty, with fair complexion, dedicate features, and grey hair. She welcomed me kindly, and conversed for a little while with a gentle, benevolent manner, but a voice that had a very sad tone in it. I found that she was a confirmed invalid, and learned afterwards that she had never recovered from the blow caused by the conduct of her husband, whom she had worshipped with real idolatry. Then we went out to see the sunset and some electrical apparatus, and on our return I was introduced to Mrs. Jameson, the authoress, who was paying a little visit, and to Dr. King, a beautiful old gentleman, more of a philosopher, however, than a physician. The next morning I had a delightful *tête-à-tête*, breakfast with Mrs. Jameson, who is a charming person with a warm Irish heart, an exquisite appreciation of art, and a deep interest in all high reform. Meanwhile it had begun to rain and the wind battered the house furiously, but nevertheless I went in the carriage with Dr. King to visit the hospital and a famous manufactory of mineral waters. I returned in a hurry to go off with Mrs. Jameson and hear Fanny Kemble read "Macbeth." This was a great treat, for I had never heard Shakespeare well given. I had caught a glimpse of Fanny Kemble the evening before, when Mrs. Jameson had brought her back from reading the "Midsummer Night's Dream." She entered the parlour for a few minutes, throwing open the door and declaiming a tragic Shakespearian quotation, dressed in rose-coloured satin, with a crimson mantle trimmed with white fur, a large bouquet in her bosom, her jet-black hair braided low down, with large black eyes, and a grand, deep-toned voice. She sat on the sofa beside Lady Byron—a most strange contrast. She was really magnificent in "Macbeth," dressed in black velvet trimmed with ermine, and Mrs. Jameson, who sat beside me, was in raptures.

The longer I saw Lady Byron the more she interested me; her insight and judgment are admirable, and I never met with a woman whose scientific tendencies seemed so strong. She seemed well versed in medicine and was her own physician, having consulted many physicians who were quite unable to aid her; she has for many years taken particular interest in labour schools, and has some admirably arranged on her estates. I much enjoyed my conversation with her, for she has a rare intelligence and a long experience. On Sunday she took me to hear a most eloquent preacher, a Mr. Robertson, who preached on the wisdom of Solomon and Christ. He is now in the Established Church, but will, I imagine, soon work himself out, for he is continually progressing, and has already drawn upon himself much persecution from his professional brethren. I certainly never heard his equal in torrent-like eloquence; it was quite a flood.

How gloriously the wind howled round the house at night! As I lay in bed and listened to the wind and the heavy swell of the waves, it was delicious. There is a pier built far out into the water as a private promenade. I had a beautiful walk there all alone one evening at sunset as the tide was coming in. On Sunday afternoon I was obliged to leave my new friends. Lady Byron, in a purple velvet mantle lined with white silk, a rich dress, and a purple satin bonnet trimmed with black lace, escorted me to the cars and put me into the second class, which economy obliged me to take. With the most hearty shake of the hand we parted, and we have exchanged several notes since I returned, for, as I said, she interests me, and I want to know more of her.

I have a standing invitation to Mrs. Jameson's Thursday evening meetings, of which I shall try to avail myself frequently. Life opens to me in London, social life particularly; but I am looking with pleasure to my return. I am too impatient to begin with my practical career to be able to stay anywhere much longer where that is not to be commenced. . . .

April 7.—Miss Murray invited me to see the Queen's favourite little German baron, but I did not accept; for to go such a distance on foot or in omnibus in my silk dress to meet people with whom I should probably have little sympathy, and to whom I should only seem a quiet, ill-dressed person, seemed to me foolish. . . . Spent the evening at Mrs. Follen's. Miss Montgomery told me a very strange story of her father's "double" appearing to her and her brother when they were children playing together during his absence in London. They were amusing themselves by dressing-up in clothes taken from a closet on the staircase, when, hearing their father's study door open and fearing reproof, they shut themselves in the closet, watching through a crack of the door their father in his dressing-gown with a candle in his hand slowly ascend the staircase. They then remembered that their father had gone to London, and rushed up to their mother's room, where she was dressing for a party, exclaiming, "Papa has come home! We saw him come out of the library with a candle in his hand and go upstairs." The authority of this story was unimpeachable, the details minute. What must one think of it? . . .

April 17.—Went down with my friend Florence to Embley Park. The laurels were in full bloom. Examined the handsome house and beautiful grounds. Saturday a perfect day. Walked much with Florence in the delicious air, amid a luxury of sights and sounds, conversing on the future. As we walked on the lawn in front of the noble drawing-room she said, "Do you know what I always think when I look at that row of windows? I think how I should turn it into a hospital ward, and just how I should place the beds!" She said she should be perfectly happy working with me, she should want no other husband.

April 20.—A beautiful Sabbath morning. Saw the sea and Isle of Wight in the distance; watched the peasants' picturesque scarlet cloaks going to church. As we crossed the fields, conversing on religious matters, it was a true communion. . . .

May 1.—A most brilliant opening of the Great Exhibition. Thanks to Cousin S., who is an exhibitor, we enjoyed a sight which we shall always remember. The place was so vast that the musical sound of the great organ was lost in the beating of the air. The great building, resplendent with the products of the whole world, was filled to overflowing with enthusiastic spectators. When the Queen, holding Prince Albert's arm, with the young Prince of Wales on one side and the Princess Royal on the other, followed by the aged Duke of Wellington arm in arm with the Marquis of Anglesea, and a long train of nobility and distinguished men, made the tour of the building and declared it open, it was indeed a memorable sight.

The advisability of remaining in England and establishing myself in practice in London was seriously considered at this time. Under other circumstances I should gladly have made the attempt, for I was strongly attracted to my native land. But I was extremely poor, with no capital to fall back on, and with a great horror of running into debt; neither had I any circle of family friends to aid me, and whilst I saw the importance of a settlement in London, I realised also its difficulties. Meanwhile the years of my study in America had produced their effect there. Popular feeling had sanctioned the effort. In both Philadelphia and Boston attempts were being made to form schools for women. My sister Emily also had adopted the medical life. She had entered the Medical College of Cleveland, Ohio, and was looking forward to joining me ultimately in the medical work; my own family also, to whom I was warmly attached, were fully expecting my return.

I determined, therefore, after much anxious consideration, to make my first settlement in New York, hoping in ten or fifteen years' time to have attained a position, when I might be able to work in England. The parting from English friends and opportunities was a painful one.

London: May 5.

I gave the day to Florence, who is about leaving, uncertain whether she will see me again. We heard Mr. Ellis lecture at the National Association on Political Economy. We also visited the Verral Hospital, but were not favourably impressed by the judiciousness of the exercises. Dined with her at the Bracebridges', and parted from her with tears.

May 20.—Visited Guy's Hospital, Dr. Oldham doing the honours most kindly. The museum is the best for study that I have yet seen. There are about 600 beds in the hospital; twenty are for midwifery, especially under Dr. Oldham's care, providing about 1,800 cases in the year, and looked after by four young students, who are maintained by the hospital for that purpose. There was a room especially devoted to electrical treatment. The whole establishment bore the marks of wealth.

July 15.—Wished Dr. Oldham good-bye, who expressed great friendliness, wished to see my sister should she visit England, and offers to make an application for admission to Guy's Hospital. . . .

July 17.—Said good-bye to Mr. Paget, Dr. Burrows, Dr. Hue, &c.—in fact, cut my connection with the hospitals. Did it with much regret; all were extremely kind, expressing the utmost interest and respect for the work. Mrs. Paget introduced me to a lady as "a benefactor to the race," and hoped to hear of me through Mr. Paget. He spoke of the perfectly satisfactory nature of the experiment, and that it may be done by another lady under similar circumstances, but *not* as a simple student, he thinks. Dr. Burrows also was extremely friendly, and paid me indirectly the highest compliment, as having "established a principle for others, by the success of my laudable enterprise; he thought that quite a new idea had been gained in this matter, which would help anyone else in future." I found also, with mingled sadness and triumph, that *now* I might do anything I pleased at St. Bartholomew's. They have learned to know and welcome me as I am going away, and are, as Mr. Paget said, sorry to lose me.

LAST DAYS IN ENGLAND—FAREWELLS

Saturday, July 19, 1851.—I have wished all good-bye, and am now ready to go. Much as I regret England, my deepest feelings are with my work, which I always carry with me. . . . Bessie P. spent part of the day with me. We parted with a few cheerful words, but I saw her face colour with emotion as she looked back and saw me watching her from the door. Beautiful, true heart! it grieves me deeply to part from her. . . .

Monday, 21st.—Left London at seven o'clock. A. turned from me in tears. I felt very sad as I looked at her thin face and thought of all she has suffered, and will suffer. . . . In the evening I met a cordial welcome at Dudley. . . . Howy and I made an expedition to Worcester and Malvern; it gave us an opportunity for much intimate conversation. We had lovely weather, and found the country exceedingly beautiful. Rode up the Worcestershire Beacon on donkeys, eating, talking, and laughing at our entanglement with other parties, and enchanted with the prospect; there was a tent on the hill, and parties dancing. We slid all the way down, and walked by Gully's and Wilson's water-cure establishments. Visited the noble old Worcester Cathedral, but looked in vain for our crest of arms, said to be there on the windows. Went over Grainger's china manufactory; the production of cups and saucers on the wheel was like magic. . . .

To Liverpool, but found the ship would not sail until Saturday. The very sight of it made me sick; so Cousin S. accompanied me to

Manchester, where we had a very interesting visit. Mr. Wilson, an intelligent business man, escorted us over a large cotton manufactory. It was of exceeding interest. Eight hundred looms were at work in one room; mostly tended by women and many very young girls. We commenced our inspection by descending by ropes deep down into the vaults, where the cotton arrives from America and India; we then proceeded through room after room where all the processes were conducted, from breaking up the bales, tearing to pieces, sorting, carding, forming into sheets, twisting, spinning, weaving, and finally measuring and folding the cloth. We went up and down, by movable trapdoors, underground from street to street, all through the immense establishment. The noise was tremendous, the dust and heat oppressive. I noticed closely the work-women, who seemed brutified by their toil; their physiognomies were assuming the projecting mouth of the lower animals. Most of them carried their hair-comb stuck in the back of their head; they were mostly youngish women, sallow and perspiring, and I noticed one woman so exhausted that she was obliged continually to sit down; they had often more than one loom to feed. They keep the men and women separate in their work as far as possible. . . .

Saturday, 26th.—Actually my last day on this noble British land! I left pale good Cousin S. standing in the street of Dudley; watched dear H. running up the railway bank as I rushed off in the train; and then I felt that I was indeed severed from England, and only anxious to get through my journey. I found myself at night on board ship, out in the Mersey. Another most important page in life fairly closed!

Adieu, dear friends! Heaven keep us all!

Chapter Five

Practical Work in America

THE first seven years of New York life were years of very difficult, though steady, uphill work. It was carried on without cessation and without change from town, either summer or winter. I took good rooms in University Place, but patients came very slowly to consult me. I had no medical companionship, the profession stood aloof, and society was distrustful of the innovation. Insolent letters occasionally came by post, and my pecuniary position was a source of constant anxiety.

Soon after settling down I made an application to be received as one of the physicians in the women's department of a large City dispensary; but the application was refused, and I was advised to form my own dispensary.

My keenest pleasure in those early days came from the encouraging letters received from the many valued English friends who extended across the ocean the warm sympathy they had shown in London. They strengthened that feeling of kinship to my native land which finally drew me back to it.

A correspondence with Lady Byron, which extended over

some years, was particularly encouraging; for the strong scientific tastes of this admirable woman, as well as her large benevolence, led her to take a steady interest in the study of medicine by women.

The following is a characteristic letter from this valued friend:—

Brighton: December 9, 1851.

I received your letter some days ago, and have ever since longed to write to you. The business which has chiefly prevented me is of a nature to interest you. A conference, originating with Miss Carpenter, is to be held at Birmingham to-morrow between chaplains, governors of gaols, magistrates, and a few ladies on the means of saving the young from sin and reforming them after its commission. I could not attend, and perhaps can render as much service in absence, indirectly. Miss Murray, Mr. Rathbone of Liverpool, Mrs. Jameson, and Miss Montgomery will be present.

The subject of this letter is to be the magnetoscope. The pamphlet by Mr. Rutter shall be sent you. Since its publication new discoveries have been made and amply tested, and of these I will try to give you some account. One objection received as conclusive against the reality of the magnetic influence from the operator was that the motions of the pendulum suspended from the instrument were produced solely by unconscious muscular movement on the part of the operator. Although to engineers and persons acquainted with the laws of motion this rotation of the pendulum in the instrument appeared to be a strange new mechanical power, yet the Royal College of Physicians and the "Lancet" decreed that it should be explained by involuntary muscular movement, and one M.D. of eminence wrote a letter to me implying that believers in the magnetoscope were to be classed with Mormons.

It has since been proved beyond a doubt by Mr. Rutter that the touch of the poles of a magnet or crystal to the spot before touched by the hand will be followed by movements exactly similar, the rotation being from east to west or from west to east, according as the north or south pole of the crystal is directed to the spot. After *contact* it occurred to Mr. R. to try *pointing only* with the poles of the crystal *held in his hand*. The same effect ensued. What becomes of the muscular impulse theory? Another objection is now considered as fatal—that when the eyes are closed all motion is stopped if the operator is either holding the thread or touching the magnetoscope. Ergo, they say, it is all imposture. But is there not another light thrown by this on the power of the eyes—on their "electric glance"? It is stated in Carpenter's "Animal Physiology" that a woman whose left arm was palsied could hold up a child with it *as long as she looked at it*. When she closed her eyes the arm dropped. A Mr. John Dimson, well known now in Brighton, has a paralytic affection of his feet, and cannot walk *unless he fixes his eyes upon them*. To this fact Mr. and Mrs. Bracebridge (Florence's friends) and Lady Easthope have recently given me their attestation as eye-witnesses, and I understand that the fact is observed at German baths for lame patients.

With the disposition, then, to "pooh-pooh" the discovery in London, I think it will probably be left to America—perhaps to you!—to evolve the truth. Therefore I shall feel it my duty to put you in possession of facts bearing upon it. I have, however, had the satisfaction of seeing conviction produced on the mind of one of our most distinguished geologists, who perceived the connection between the influences of magnetism and metals on the pendulum, and some of the subterranean operations, particularly mineral springs. (My hand is tired and must rest.)

The application of magnetism to the principle of life is most satisfactory to me. The unification of the magnetism of the human head by finding that the pendulum is influenced by it, exactly as by a real magnet, that the poles correspond, the forehead being north when the person is upright. (Changes take place in the recumbent position.) This is when a person stands in any direction, *live* bodies being *independently* magnetic. It is the case even with an egg new laid. After boiling, *that* power ceases, and it is a magnet only *by induction*, like any other inorganic matter. In trying experiments the feet must not be crossed, nor the legs, nor the hands clasped, nor thumbs joined. These attitudes all occasion the motions to stop—for they complete this circuit—analogous to electrical phenomena. After all, I have not told you what appears the most curious fact in its consequences, that (as far as yet tried) the body loses its influence on the magnetoscope in sleep. Its polarity is gone, as in death! "Twin brothers!"

On reading over what I have written I perceive a want of explicitness, which I hope the pamphlet will make up. I will divide it into sheets to be sent in letters.

With a strong feeling that the ocean is not distance,

Yours most truly,

A. I. NOEL BYRON.

At this time I employed the leisure hours of a young physician in preparing some lectures on the physical education of girls, which were delivered in a basement Sunday school room in the spring of 1852.

These lectures, owing to the social and professional connections which resulted from them, gave me my first start in practical medical life. They were attended by a small but very intelligent audience of ladies, and amongst them were some members of the Society of Friends, whose warm and permanent interest was soon enlisted. Indeed, my practice during those early years became very much a Quaker practice; and the institutions which sprang up later owed their foundation to the active support of this valuable section of the community. The family of Mr. Stacy B. Collins, a highly respected member of the Society of Friends, will always be affectionately remembered. They first engaged me as the family physician. The granddaughter, now Dr. Mary B. Hussey, was my "first baby"; and a warm friendship continues into the third generation. The names also of Robert Haydock, Merritt Trimble, and Samuel Willets will always be gratefully remembered in connection with this movement in New York. These well-known and highly respected citizens with their families gradually became our most steadfast friends.

My first medical consultation was a curious experience. In a severe case of pneumonia in an elderly lady I called in consultation a kind-hearted physician of high standing who had been present in Cincinnati at the time of my father's fatal illness. This gentleman, after seeing the patient, went with me into the parlour. There he began to walk about the room in some agitation, exclaiming, "A most extraordinary case! Such a one never happened to me before; I really do not know what to do!" I listened in surprise and much perplexity, as it was a clear case of pneumonia and of no unusual degree of danger, until at last I discovered that his perplexity related to *me*, not to the patient, and to the propriety of consulting with a lady physician! I was both amused and relieved. I at once assured my old acquaintance that it need not be considered in the light of an ordinary consultation, if he were uneasy about it, but as a friendly talk. So, finally, he gave me his best advice; my patient rapidly got well, and happily I never afterwards had any difficulty in obtaining a necessary consultation from members of the profession.

In 1852, warmly encouraged by Mrs. Dr. Bellows, I published the lectures I had given, under the title, "The Laws of Life in reference to the Physical Education of Girls." This little work was favourably regarded by physicians; it drew forth an encouraging letter from the dean of my college, to my very great gratification. It also happened to fall under Mr. Ruskin's notice, and gained his valuable commendation.

Being still excluded from medical companionship, and from the means of increasing medical knowledge which dispensary practice affords, I finally determined to try and form an independent dispensary.

In 1853, with the aid of some of my friends, a small room was engaged in a poor quarter of the town near Tompkin's Square; one of my Quaker friends, Mrs. Cornelia Hussey, actively assisted in arranging drugs, covering a screen, &c. This dispensary (afterwards moved to Third Street) was opened three afternoons in each week, and I had the satisfaction during the following two years of finding it welcomed by the poor, and steadily enlisting a larger circle of friends.

In 1854 the Act of Incorporation for an institution where women physicians could be available for the poor was obtained, and a few well-known citizens consented to act as trustees. The first annual report of this modest little dispensary is given in the Appendix. From this very small beginning have gradually arisen the present flourishing institutions of the New York Infirmary and College for Women.

It was during these first early years that, not being able to continue the expense of good consultation-rooms, I determined to *buy* a house. A friend lent me the necessary money at fair interest, and a house in a good situation in Fifteenth Street was selected. This transaction proved a very material assistance in many different ways, and enabled me to form the home center which is so necessary to the most efficient work. In later years also this early experience helped me to realise more fully the fundamental importance of the great land question, or "a stake in the soil," as well as other weighty social problems.

The difficulties and trials encountered at this early period were severe. Ill-natured gossip, as well as insolent anonymous letters, came to me. Although I have never met with any serious difficulties in attending to my practice at all hours of the night, yet unpleasant annoyances from unprincipled men were not infrequent. Some well-dressed man would walk by my side on Broadway, saying in a low voice, "Turn down Duane Street to the right"; or whilst waiting for a horse-car at midnight by the City Hall a policeman would try to take my hand; or a group of late revellers would shout across the street, "See that lone woman walking like mad!" But with common sense, self-reliance, and attention to the work in hand, any woman can pursue the medical calling without risk.

The heat of a New York summer also was at this time very trying to an English constitution. A letter to my sister in 1853 exclaims:—

> Oh, dear! it is so hot I can hardly write. I was called this morning to Flushing to see a sick child, and then attended my dispensary, the thermometer varying from 86 to 90 in the house, and it stood at 102 in some rooms down town. Walk as deliberately as I would, it made my brain seem too large for my head. Flushing reminded me of the Sahara; it lay breathless under a cloudless sky, leaden with haze.

In relation to mischievous gossip it is written:—

These malicious stories are painful to me, for I am woman as well as physician, and both natures are wounded by these falsehoods. Ah, I am glad I, and not another, have to bear this pioneer work. I understand now why this life has never been lived before. It *is* hard, with no support but a high purpose, to live against every species of social opposition. . . . I *should* like a little fun now and then. Life is altogether too sober.

The utter loneliness of life became intolerable, and in October of 1854 I took a little orphan girl from the great emigrant depôt of Randall's Island to live with me. This congenial child I finally adopted. The wisdom of such adoption is abundantly shown by an entry in my journal, two years later, written on my birthday:—

On this bright Sunday morning I feel full of hope and strength for the future. Kitty plays beside me with her doll. She has just given me a candy basket, purchased with a penny she had earned, full of delight in "Doctor's birthday"! Who will ever guess the restorative support which that poor little orphan has been to me? When I took her to live with me she was about seven and a half years old. I desperately needed the change of thought she compelled me to give her. It was a dark time, and she did me good—her genial, loyal, Irish temperament suited me. Now I look forward with much hope to the coming events of this year.

An amusing circumstance relating to this child is worth recording. She had always been accustomed to call me "Doctor." On one occasion she was present during the visit of a friendly physician. After he was gone, she came to me with a very puzzled face, exclaiming, "Doctor, how very odd it is to hear a *man* called Doctor!"

In December of 1855 I gave a first drawing-room "Address on the Medical Education of Women."

In this address (which was afterwards printed) it was shown that the movement was only a revival of work in which women had always been engaged; but that it was a revival in an advanced form, suited to the age and to the enlarging capabilities of women.

The clear perception of the providential call to women to take their full share in human progress has always led us to insist upon a full and identical medical education for our students. From the beginning in America, and later on in England, we have always refused to be tempted by the specious offers urged upon us to be satisfied with partial or specialised instruction. On the occasion of this address an appeal was made for assistance in collecting funds for the growth of the dispensary and the gradual formation of a hospital, as indispensable for the accomplishment of the work. A committee of three ladies was appointed at this drawing-room meeting, for the purpose of beginning the difficult work of collecting a permanent fund.

In 1854, my sister, Dr. Emily Blackwell, who had graduated with honour at the Medical College of Cleveland, Ohio, was pursuing her studies in Europe.

There she gained invaluable surgical experience from having been generously received as assistant by Sir James Simpson in his extensive practice in female diseases. The genial character of this well-known physician was shown not only by his cordial reception of Dr. Emily as pupil and assistant, but by an amusing incident which occurred whilst his consulting-rooms were filled by a waiting assembly of aristocratic patients. My sister, being a classical scholar, was often employed by the Doctor in making translations or extracts for him. On one occasion, whilst thus engaged in the farthest room of the suite, he called in a low voice, "Dr. Blackwell," then a little louder, "*Dr. Blackwell*," and when the attention of all his patients was thus aroused, he called in a voice loud enough for my sister to hear, "Dr. BLACKWELL!" and then from the corner of his eye, and with intense amusement, he watched the varied expressions of surprise and dismay depicted on the countenances of his distinguished patients as they saw the approach along the suite of rooms of a lady who thus answered to the summons.

The following letters to my medical sister refer to this period of the work:—

New York: May 12.

I need not tell you with what interest and hope I look forward to your Edinburgh news. The prospect is very good. . . . One of the most difficult points I have to contend with here is the entire absence of medical sympathy; the medical solitude is really awful at times; I should thankfully turn to any educated woman if I could find one. . . . Pray bear in mind to collect all the information you can about maternity, the relation of the sexes, and kindred subjects. We have a vast field to work in this direction, for reliable information is desperately needed in the world on these topics. I feel as if it were peculiarly our duty to meet this want. There is much vain thought given to these matters here. An active set of people are making desperate efforts to spread their detestable doctrines of "free love" under scientific guise, placing agents with the advertisements of their books worded in the most specious and attractive manner at the doors of the conventions now being held here; on the other hand, equally misleading publications are brought out in opposition. Such teaching is utterly superficial and untrustworthy, and consequently misleading. We want facts, scientifically accurate observations, past and present, on all that bears on these matters. . . .

You remember the pamphlet sent me by Dr. Sims of Alabama. He is now here, determined to establish a hospital for the special treatment of women's diseases; he is enlisting much support, and will, I think, succeed. He seems to be in favour of women studying medicine. I think I shall help him in any way I can. . . .

I have at last found a student in whom I can take a great deal of interest—Marie Zackrzewska, a German, about twenty-six. Dr. Schmidt, the head of the Berlin midwifery department, discovered her talent, advised her to study, and finally appointed her as chief midwife in the hospital under him; there she taught classes of about 150 women and 50 young men, and proved herself most capable. When Dr. Schmidt died, the American Minister advised her to come to New York; but here the German doctors wanted her to become a nurse. In desperation she consulted "The Home for the Friendless," where they advised her to come to me. There is true stuff in her, and I shall do my best to bring it out. She must obtain a medical degree. . . .

July 24.

Don't be discouraged. There is no doubt about our losing many opportunities because of our sex, but you must also bear in mind the disadvantages all students labour under, unless in exceptional cases. Crowded together in masses, they only see at a distance the most interesting cases; the complete study is reserved for the physician or his constant attendant. I remember expressing my impatience while in the Maternité at the restrictive rules there, and M. Blot said, "What you wish for are only enjoyed by the few who occupy the most favoured positions." Yet I gained, in spite of all difficulties, a great deal, and in accelerating ratio the longer I stayed. I remember that it seemed to me

I had gained more in my fourth month at the Maternité than in the whole three preceding ones. Now I say this because I don't want you to over-estimate the worth of pantaloons. Disguise in France or elsewhere would by no means give you all you need; if the disguise were complete you would just be reduced to the level of the common poor student, and would be, I think, quite disappointed. It needs also that influential men should take an interest in you, and give you chances quite beyond the ordinary run. I know that at St. Bartholomew's I would not have exchanged my position for that of the simple student, though I would gladly for the clinical clerk or *interne's* position. Now you can do nothing in France, except by special medical influence. Your time is limited, and you cannot wait for examinations and promotions as an ordinary student. You ask me what I did, and what can be done as a lady. I entered the Maternité, dissected at l'Ecole des Beaux-Arts alone, employed a *répétiteur* who drilled me in anatomy and smuggled me into the dead-house of La Charité at great risk of detection, where I operated on the *cadavre.* I once made the rounds of his wards in the Hôtel-Dieu with Roux, heard his lectures, and saw his operations. I attended lectures on medical generalities at the College of France and Jardin des Plantes. I believe that was all in the way of Parisian study. I applied to Davenne, Director-General of the hospitals, for permission to follow the physicians—refused; applied to Dubois and Trousseau to attend lectures at the Ecole de Médecine—refused; Trousseau advising me to disguise. You see I had no introductions, no experience. I went into the Maternité soon after going to France, and came out with a sad accident, not inclined to renew the battle, not well knowing how, and with a promising chance opened to me in London. I should do differently now. I should get the most influential introduction I could; I should tell them just what I wanted, find which hospitals would be most suited to my purpose, and if by putting on disguise I could get either an assistant's post or good visiting privilege, I would put it on. I don't believe it would be a disguise at all to those you were thrown with, but it would be a protection if advised by intelligent men, and would make them free to help you. I should avoid crowds, because you gain nothing in them; I don't think either the lectures at l'Ecole de Médecine or the great hospital visits, where from one to five hundred students follow, would be of any use. It is in a more private and intimate way, and in hospitals where many students do not go, that you might gain. I know no one in a position to give you more valuable letters than Dr. Simpson, if he is disposed to. You ask me what I saw at the Maternité, but I find my notes imperfect; I have only noted down nine versions, &c. But I think the most important thing in the Maternité is the drilling in the more ordinary labours, for only where the finger is thoroughly trained can you detect varieties. The cases you send me are very interesting, and I am very glad you have made such full notes, as they will be useful hints in future solitary practice. Don't be in a hurry to leave Dr. S., for I fear you will nowhere else find a good drilling in that department. I shall see how far I can make your notes available from time to time in my own practice. With regard to my own *clientèle*, I shall have advanced 50 dollars over last year; slow progress, but still satisfactory, as it is reliable practice, not capricious success. Only think, the thermometer has been up to 102 in some of the rooms down town! We have had three days' "spells" this July that seem to me a little beyond anything I have ever had to endure.

November 13.

I shall be very anxious to know what you do in Paris. I almost doubt the propriety of your entering the Maternité, or rather I hope that the necessity may be obviated by your finding other openings. That Dubois is somewhat of an old fox, and will, I presume, at once advise your entrance, to get rid of any responsibility; but I would not think of doing so until I had seen all the others and tried for better openings. I think you could get sufficient midwifery at the Ecole de Médecine, where the midwives have the night cases; the association would be unpleasant from the character of the women, but it would leave you your freedom. You have done excellently in Edinburgh, and nothing could be more satisfactory than the way you leave. I think, however, before going to Paris you had certainly better see Dr. Oldham of Guy's; he is disposed to be friendly, and if he chose might greatly help you. It would seem as if it would be well to pursue your English studies before the Parisian; if you could follow Doctors Burrows and Baly in medicine at St. Bartholomew's, and Oldham at Guy's, you would do well. I am very glad you are collecting special medical statistics; we shall find them very serviceable in lecture or pamphlet form. It will be necessary next year to make an active effort for the dispensary, and I think a few lectures would be very important. My conviction becomes constantly stronger that you will return, and my plans for the future all involve that fact. A pleasant circumstance occurred to my German, Dr. Zackrzewska. I arranged a Cleveland course for her, and she entered two weeks ago; she met a very friendly reception, and found that Dr. Kirkland is in correspondence with Professor Müller of Berlin, and he had mentioned her in some of his letters in such high terms, that the faculty told her, if she would qualify herself for examination in surgery and chemistry and write an English thesis, that they would graduate her at the end of this term. Of course she is studying with might and main, and will, I have no doubt, succeed; so we may reckon on a little group of three next year. That will be quite encouraging.

November 27.

I cannot but feel glad that you rejected the urgent persuasions to go to the Crimea. I cannot say what going to Russia might have done for you in *English* reputation, but for America it would have been sheer waste of time. I am constantly surprised to see what an entire non-conductor of enthusiasm the ocean is, and reputation in England, except in very rare cases, is utterly unavailing here. The radical differences in national character, and the eager, youthful nature of this people, quite prevent full sympathetic transmission of feeling and recognition of older experience. I am vexed to think how completely unavailing your Scotch studies will be in the *puffing* line, but make yourself really strong, and we will turn them to the best account in another and a better way. Don't forget to bring a full earnest testimonial from Simpson and from others as you progress.

I'm delighted you are going to Malvern. Oh, those breezy uplands of our native isle! is anything in Nature so delicious as their air and freedom? My ride with K. over the Welsh hills stands alone in my memory, and my slide with Howy down Malvern makes my mouth water.

January 23, 1855.

Your letter came yesterday, giving me an account of M.'s relapse and the many anxieties you have suffered lately. I confess to feeling an intense anxiety about her notwithstanding the hope conveyed in your letter, and I shall look to the coming of the postman with dread for the next three weeks lest he should bring me evil news. You have been pursuing your studies in a way we did not anticipate the last eight weeks, but very surely it is not lost time; the responsibilities of such a case will strengthen you for every future case, and as an illustration of or commentary on Dr. S.'s practice, I don't think it will be lost to you. The whole case from beginning to end strikes me as a horrid barbarism, but at the same time I fully allow that it is the way to make a reputation. M.'s death would be little to him, the responsibility would be staved off in a dozen different ways, and if she succeeded in her object, no end to the trumpeting of his praise! I see every day that it is the "heroic," self-reliant, and actively *self-imposing* practitioner that excites a sensation and reputation; the rational and conscientious physician is not the famous one.

I have just heard one piece of news which decidedly indicates progress and which is peculiarly cheering to me, because I am persuaded that I have been chiefly instrumental in it. The New York Hospital has opened its doors to women this winter; there is now a class of eight women, all pupils from Dr. Trail's hydropathic institute, who attend regularly the clinical visits and lectures in the amphitheatre with all the other students. The matter was discussed in full board, Trimble and Collins both advocating, and it was resolved to make the experiment, Drs. Smith, Buck, and Watson, the then attending physicians, being present and consenting, quite concurring in the principle, and only pleading the embarrassment they should themselves occasionally feel. Mr. Trimble assured them they would soon conquer their bashfulness! Thus far, it seems, there has been no difficulty. I consider the matter so important that I intend at once to take the hospital ticket and watch the experiment in person as closely as I can. I only wish the girls came from other than quack auspices.

Do the "knockings" prevail at all in England? it is astonishing how they increase here. Judge Edmunds has published two large volumes, which are astonishing, I think, as a record of self-deception or credulity. The promoters hold public discussions in the tabernacle, publish endless literature, and have hired a large house in Broadway at 2,200 dollars, and Katy Fox at a salary of 1,200 dollars per annum to give free demonstrations to whoever wishes to investigate the truth of "this wonderful new revelation." I attended one of these free sittings lately at Mrs. B.'s invitation. It was a curious physical phenomenon to my mind of the animal magnetism order. My few questions were all answered wrong; but Mrs. B. and many others asked similar questions, the answers of which she knew, and they were answered promptly and correctly. Everyone who queried with eager temperament got prompt and correct replies, independent of Katy Fox's volition. It was odd, but quite disgusting in the view taken of it, as an ultra-mundane exhibition.

Establishment of a hospital.—In 1856 my working powers were more than doubled by the arrival of my sister, Dr. Emily Blackwell, who became henceforth my partner and able co-worker. Dr. Maria E. Zackrzewska also joined us as soon as she had graduated at Cleveland, and became for some years before her removal to Boston our active and valued assistant in the New York work.

The refreshing Sunday walks taken with this warm-hearted doctor when, crossing the bay by an early ferry-boat, we walked for hours in the beautiful environs of Hoboken or Staten Island, will always remain as a pleasant background to the affectionate friendship which still continues.

Thus reinforced, an advanced step was made in 1857 by the renting of a house, No. 64 Bleecker Street, which we fitted up for a hospital where both patients and young assistant physicians could be received. This institution, under the name of "The New York Infirmary for Women and Children," was formally opened in the May of this year by a public meeting, in which the Rev. Henry Ward Beecher, Dr. Elder of Philadelphia, and the Rev. Dr. Tyng, jun., warmly supported the movement. In this institution Dr. Zackrzewska accepted the post of resident physician, Dr. Emily becoming chiefly responsible for the surgical practice.

This first attempt to establish a hospital conducted entirely by women excited much opposition. At that date, although college instruction was being given to women students in some places, no hospital was anywhere available either for practical instruction or the exercise of the woman-physician's skill. To supply the need had become a matter of urgent importance. Our difficulties are thus noted in the Annual Report for 1864:—

"But to this step (the establishment of a hospital) a host of objections were raised by those whom the early friends of the institution attempted to interest in their effort. They were told that no one would let a house for the purpose, that female doctors would be looked upon with so much suspicion that the police would interfere; that if deaths occurred their death certificates would not be recognised; that they would be resorted to by classes and persons whom it would be an insult to be called upon to deal with; that without men as resident physicians they would not be able to control the patients; that if any accident occurred, not only the medical profession but the public would blame the trustees for supporting such an undertaking; and, finally, that they would never be able to collect money enough for so unpopular an effort."

Through a cloud of discouragement and distrust the little institution steadily worked its way, its few friends holding to it the more firmly for the difficulties it experienced. The practice of the infirmary, both medical and surgical, was conducted entirely by women; but a board of consulting physicians, men of high standing in the profession, gave it the sanction of their names. Dr. Valentine Mott, Dr. John Watson, Drs. Willard Parker, R. S. Kissam, Isaac E. Taylor, and George P. Camman were the earliest medical friends of the infirmary.

The pecuniary support of this institution, in addition to the medical responsibility involved in its conduct, was no small burden. For many years its annual income rested mainly on our exertions. A bazaar was held in its behalf for seven years in succession; lectures, concerts, and every other available means of collecting funds were resorted to.

At one time Fanny Kemble was giving a series of Shakespearian readings in New York, and often rendered generous help to benevolent institutions by the use of her great talent. We hoped that she might aid our struggling infirmary by giving a public reading in its behalf. So on one occasion I called with our fellow-worker Dr. Zackrzewska at the hotel where she was staying to prefer our request. She received us courteously, listened with kindness to an explanation of the object of our visit and of the needs of the infirmary; but when she heard that the physicians of the institution were *women* she sprang up to her full height, turned her flashing eyes upon us, and with the deepest tragic tones of her magnificent voice exclaimed: "Trust a *woman*—as a DOCTOR!—NEVER!"

The thunder-clap which thus smote us in the New York hotel brought back amusingly to my mind the scene at Brighton, when the parlour door suddenly opened, and a brilliant figure in stage costume advanced to the gentle, refined Lady Byron with an impassioned quotation from "Julius Cæsar." The contrast between two women's natures was so remarkable!

The necessity, however, of a separate hospital for the general training of women students had by this time been recognised. Experience both at the New York Hospital and at the large Bellevue Hospital, where classes of imperfectly trained women had failed to maintain their ground, proved that a special woman's centre was needed, not only as affording them practical instruction, but for the purpose of testing the capacity and tact of the students themselves, before admitting them to walk the general hospitals where male students were admitted. The New York Infirmary for Women therefore gradually enlisted the active help of enlightened men and women.

We were much encouraged by the kindly contributions of articles for our annual bazaars from English friends; and a generous-hearted French lady, Madame Trélat, who felt much interest in the new medical movement sent a donation to the funds of the hospital. The continued interest of English friends is shown by our correspondence.

TO LADY NOEL BYRON

New York: December 27, 1857.

MY DEAR FRIEND,—Your kind interest in our hospital cheers me. Very few persons understand the soul of this work, or the absolute necessity which lies upon us to live out the ideal life to the utmost of our power. My work is undoubtedly for the few. It is labour in the inter-linkings of humanity, and is necessarily difficult of appreciation by the mass of people, and is very slow in gaining their esteem. It has been a most toilsome lesson to translate my thought into the common language of life. I labour at this translation perpetually, and still remain too often incomprehensible. I will not degrade the central thought of this work, but I seek in every way to accommodate it wisely to the practical common-sense feeling of the people.

My sister is a noble helper, and we shall stand, I trust, shoulder to shoulder through many years of active service. I shall have the pleasure of soon forwarding to you a report of our last year's proceedings; this will give the simple facts of our hospital life.

Allow me to remain, with very true affection,

Your friend,

ELIZABETH BLACKWELL.

79 East Fifteenth Street.

Chapter Six

England Revisited

1858

THE ten years during which this pioneer medical work had been steadily carried on had thus firmly established the new departure as a useful innovation in the United States. The reform was at that time steadily growing, not only in New York, but also in Philadelphia and Boston, under the guidance of able bodies of women. We were now desirous of learning what openings existed in England for the entrance of women into the medical profession. We knew that much interest had been felt there in the progress of the American work, and we had been urged by friends in Europe to give some account of it.

It was determined, therefore, in August 1858 that I should again revisit my native land and urge the importance of this medical work. Soon after my arrival in Europe I took the occasion of a visit made to a sister in Paris to prepare carefully a series of three addresses to be delivered in England, showing what was being done in medicine by women in the United States, and the reasons for that work. The first of these addresses was on the value of physiological knowledge to women, the second on the value of medical knowledge, and the third on the practical aspect of the work as established in America and its adaptability to England. Whilst engaged in the preparation of the lectures I entered into relations with the large-hearted Countess de Noailles, whose devotion to sanitary reform and generous support of benevolent enterprises were equally remarkable. This lady was very desirous that a country sanatorium for women should be established in England or France, being firmly convinced that hygienic conditions in their fullest application were the chief necessity in the successful treatment of special diseases. This lady wrote to an old friend in Paris: "I wish to direct all my efforts to this object. Let me know as soon as possible what it would cost to establish a small hospital for women and children either in France or England, under Miss Blackwell's direction." She also requested one of her noble French relatives to make my acquaintance. The interview is thus described in a letter to Dr. Emily in New York.

Paris: 1858.

Yesterday I saw Madame—by appointment at her own house. A. says she is a daughter of the Prince de P.; to me she seemed a stout, black-eyed Frenchwoman of forty-five, cordial in manner, speaking English well, and knowing as much of England and Anglo-Saxon nature as a French-woman ever can know. We conversed energetically for two hours. She is seriously interested in the entrance of women into the medical profession, a wish founded in her case on the moral degradation which she has observed amongst her own acquaintance from the practice of being treated by men in female complaints. The fact which most struck her in all I told her was your amputating a breast; in this she actually triumphed. Her face became radiant with the intense satisfaction of the thing, for it proved to her by a fact what she wanted to believe, but could only accept intellectually from all my reasons—viz. the necessity of letting the midwife drop, and striking unflinchingly for the highest position. This one fact, worth to this sort of nature a host of arguments, gave her real faith in the physician. She opened freely her objections, or rather difficulties, and I met them one after another; and this difference I observed in the encounter with the cultivated European nature—when I gave her a reason she understood it and accepted it; it did not go in at one ear and out at the other as with more frivolous people; there is some soil or substance you can plant in in this stouter nature. As years ago with Lady Byron, so with this lady, it was of some use talking to her. She propounded, of course, foolish as well as serious ideas; thus she thought that women physicians should never marry; she also would be shocked to see me with a garland on my head dancing in a ballroom, and she thought they should be devoted, like the sisters of charity, &c. I combated her idea of abnegation for a while, and put in a feeler to see if she could take in a higher notion; but finding it was impossible, I at once ceased the attempt, and allowed her to hold to her own highest idea, which I could see was tinged by her French nature. Of course it wearied me a little, and I wanted after a while to expand my lungs and breathe freely; but I certainly made a strong impression upon her. She thanked me and shook my hand again and again at parting, and said that she should not think of letting this be our last interview, and she should write to Madame de Noailles the very next day. She had asked me previously if I was resolved in any case to go back to America, and I had told her "No," but described at the same time the excellent beginning we had made there. I feel convinced that I shall have some proposition in relation to my (or rather our) establishment in London. What, then, ought we to say should such an offer arise? I will accept nothing that is not offered to us both, on that I am quite determined; we cannot separate in practice.

Paris: November, 1858.

Preparing my lectures is a troublesome business. My first one would not do; it was so much more adapted to an American than an English audience. I wanted also quantities of facts that I did not know how to get. But I have now re-written twenty-one pages. I have written it with pleasure, though very slowly, and I am really surprised to find how very slowly I write. I can only write when I feel fresh in the morning; sometimes only a page, sometimes none. I will not force it when I don't feel fresh, but I shall take whatever time is necessary to do the work well, for it is really important.

It was during this visit that I had the privilege of becoming personally acquainted with Dr. Trélat, the head of La Salpêtrière, and his admirable wife, who remained steadfast friends through life. I visited them at La Salpêtrière—that large asylum for infirm women, over which Dr. Trélat presided with truly paternal care. La Salpêtrière was not then a great school of experimentation, but a benevolent refuge, where the well-being and kindly protection of its inmates formed the primary object of the director.

The following letters are descriptive of this time.

TO LADY BYRON

Paris: December 30, 1858.
160 Rue St. Dominique.

MY DEAR AND VENERATED FRIEND,—I received your letter yesterday. The mere chance of being in any way useful to the valuable friend you refer to is reason sufficient for a short return at once to England, so I have made my arrangements to reach London on Monday evening, January 3.

I have heard with great pleasure of an invitation to lecture in London, which I will acknowledge when I receive it. I shall be glad of an opportunity of laying very important considerations before my fellow country-women, but I cannot lecture just at present. I find that I must first go to Italy, for reasons which I will explain when we meet; therefore it is too soon to engage rooms at present, for which kind offer I sincerely thank you.

My chief object in making this hurried visit of a few days is to see Miss Nightingale and a few valued friends, amongst whom I hope I may reckon yourself. I shall therefore remain quietly at my cousin's, No. 73 Gloucester Terrace, Hyde Park, not attempting to enter into society.

TO DR. EMILY BLACKWELL

London: February 1859.

I have just returned from an interview with Miss Nightingale at Malvern in relation to a school for nurses which she wishes to establish; and I start to-morrow for France *en route*, for Mentone. My old friend's health is failing from the pressure of mental labour. I cannot go into the details of her last five years now, but the labour has been and is immense. I think I have never known a woman labour as she has done. It is a most remarkable experience; she indeed deserves the name of a worker. Of course we conversed very earnestly about the nursing plan in which she wished to interest me. She says that for six months she shall be utterly unable to give any thought to the fund work, and wants me meanwhile to observe English life very carefully, and make up my mind as to whether I can give up America, which she thinks a very serious matter. Unfortunately she does not think private practice possible in connection with her plan. If so, it would be impossible for us to help her. She thinks her own health will never permit her to carry out her plan herself, and I much fear she is right in this belief.

After a short visit to the Riviera, to confer with the Countess de Noailles about her proposed sanatorium for women, I returned to London. There my warm friends the Misses Leigh Smith, supported by their generous-hearted father, and Miss Bessie Rayner Parkes, interested themselves actively in preparing for the first delivery of my lectures. The Marylebone Hall was secured. Our young friends brought up primroses and other lovely flowers and green wreaths from Hastings to ornament the reading-desk, and warmly supported me by their ardent sympathy. On March 2, 1859, the first lecture was given to a very intelligent and appreciative audience, whose interest was warmly enlisted. I well remember the tears rolling down the benevolent face of Miss Anna Goldsmid, who sat immediately in front of me. But the most important listener was the bright, intelligent young lady whose interest in the study of medicine was then aroused—Miss Elizabeth Garrett—who became the pioneer of the medical movement in England, and who, as Mrs.

Garrett Anderson, lives to see the great success of her difficult and brave work.

These addresses were afterwards given in Manchester, Birmingham, and Liverpool; Mr. Bracebridge kindly making arrangements for them in Birmingham and the Rev. W. H. Channing in Liverpool.

The interest thus excited in London led to some effort being made to commence in England similar work to that being done in America. A meeting of ladies was held at the St. John's Wood residence of Mrs. Peter Taylor, over which Mr. William Shaen presided. A committee was formed to consider the subject, and encouraged by the offer of help made by the Countess de Noailles, a circular was prepared, stating the object to be accomplished and inviting support. This circular, which was revised by Dr. Mayo, Lady Byron, Mr. Shaen, and the Hon. Russell Gurney, was gradually signed by a large number of influential ladies.

[Circular.]

PROPOSED HOSPITAL FOR THE TREATMENT OF THE SPECIAL DISEASES OF WOMEN

THE Lectures recently delivered by Doctor Elizabeth Blackwell at the Marylebone Literary Institution have produced in the minds of the ladies who heard them a strong conviction of the necessity for a more general diffusion of hygienic knowlege among women; and have led to a proposition to found a hospital for a class of diseases, the ordinary treatment of which too frequently involves much avoidable moral suffering, to be placed under the direction of competent women physicians, in connection with a Board of consulting physicians and surgeons.

A lady, impressed with the want of such an institution, and convinced of the value of hygienic knowledge in the treatment and prevention of female diseases, has already promised 1,000*l*. towards the hospital, and offers 5,000*l*. more for the endowment of a Sanitary Professorship in connection with it, provided a sufficient sum be raised by donation to place the institution on a permanent basis.

In order to secure the advantages of this offer, it is proposed to raise and invest an additional sum of not less than 10,000*l*. for the purpose of securing and furnishing a suitable house, and forming the nucleus of a permanent hospital endowment; and also to collect an annual subscription list of not less than 500*l*., to assist in defraying the current expenses of the hospital.

The ladies whose names are appended to this statement have signified their cordial concurrence in the proposal to establish such an institution, and their desire to aid it in any way that may be within their power.

Contributions will be received by Messrs. Williams, Deacon & Co., Bankers, 20 Birchin Lane, E.C. Any communications may be addressed to Miss Braysher, Hon. Secretary, 73 Gloucester Terrace, Hyde Park, W.

Messrs. Bracebridge, the Hon. Russell Gurney, Q.C., and the Hon. W. Cowper accepted the posts of trustees, and sixty-six names of well-known ladies were gradually added to the circular.

TO DR. EMILY BLACKWELL, NEW YORK

London: April 15, 1859.

The more I see of work in England, the more I like it. From the Queen downwards I see signs of favour. On all hands we make converts, and those who are indoctrinated make converts. The whole way in which the cause is regarded by laity and doctors is most respectful. I believe we could get into general practice. We could shape the whole matter in the right way, for people welcome true ideas. There is an immense charm in this fresh field, where solid English heads receive the highest view of truth, where generosity and largeness of idea meet you at every turn. I like working and living in England, and there is no limit to what we might accomplish here. But, alas! there is the same old difficulty. We ought to have an independent 300*l.* per annum between us, and for want of that it is all vitiated. I see the charm of work here as clearly as I did on my arrival nine months ago, and feel immeasurably more hopeful about the possibilities of English work, but I realise more than ever the difficulty of working here upon nothing. I am writing to you upon our last prospectus, one which is to be widely circulated when we are satisfied with the names appended. It has been carefully revised, and it is contemplated to distribute many thousands of them. But we have been six weeks shaping the prospectus and collecting some names, and I know that it will take many weeks more to secure the names it is hoped to obtain. In fact, it is a long work of initiation that has to be carried on, which would be very thorough, excellently well done, but which I cannot wait to do.

It is very unfortunate that the probable dissolution of Parliament and consequent ferment of re-elections will interfere with our proceedings; all lecturing is out of the question during the excitement of elections.

I shall probably join A. in the Isle of Wight for a week or two. I do want to see that dear little island again, and I shall there find leisure to revise my little book for an English edition.

I am going to dine with the Gurneys to-night, to meet the Rev. Mr. Maurice, who is so highly regarded by a large party, and whom I am to convert! It will be a clerical party to-night, and to-morrow I am engaged to meet a few medical gentlemen at Mr. Hawes's!

The country looks lovely, and as usual I am longing for it, and will break away at Easter for a little holiday. How hard you must be working! You must have a holiday when I come back.

Easter was spent in the Isle of Wight revising the little work on "The Laws of Life," an English edition of which was brought out by Sampson Low & Co.

During this time the plan of the proposed hospital was being circulated in London.

It was during this visit to England that the important step was taken of placing a woman's name on the authorised Medical Register of the United Kingdom. Influential friends were desirous of keeping me in England. They presented the various testimonials of English and Continental study given by distinguished physicians and credentials of American practice to the Medical Council. On this council, of which Sir Benjamin Brodie was president, were old friends of the St. Bartholomew's days. The subject was very carefully considered, and after mature deliberation this just and important concession to qualified women was authorised. I had the satisfaction of being enrolled as a recognised physician of my native land in the Medical Register of January 1, 1859.

TO DR. EMILY BLACKWELL, NEW YORK

May 13, 1859.

My letter this week must be rather short, for I am overwhelmed with all sorts of engagements previous to leaving for Birmingham, where I give my first provincial lecture next Monday. I have communicated to our little committee Madame de Noailles's insistence upon a country site for the hospital, and also the necessity that exists for not abandoning our work in New York until the institutions there are self-supporting. They are very much disappointed by the country condition attached to the hospital; but were I settled in England and working there, it would not discourage them. But all our friends seem to think that as the New York Infirmary is the best argument that can be used for English work, its downfall would be an irreparable misfortune, and they are willing, under the circumstances, to let me go. Indeed, I find it necessary to come to a decision myself, and after carefully weighing everything I have made up my mind to return, at any rate for some time. I can secure any amount of personal interest from various quarters; but as the prospect of speedily realising an institution where we could both work is put farther off, I do not wish to stay under the circumstances. . . .

Edgbaston: May 17,1859.

A letter just received from the Countess de Noailles urges me to begin a sanatorium in the country near New York. She says: "As the central hospital already exists in New York, if you will allow me to help in beginning a sanatorium in country air I should be able to realise my idea at once. I think you might obtain some house or farm-house for the purpose in the course of the autumn or spring. The importance of convalescent hospitals in the country is beginning to be recognised in England; let women be the first to set the example of one in America. I believe that in women's complaints they are of more importance than in any other, and that in seven cases out of ten the air alone would effect the cure." Now I think this is extremely rational and liberal, and we must discuss together how we can do it for her.

TO LADY BYRON

73 Gloucester Terrace, Hyde Park: June 10, 1859.

It grieves me much to know of these constantly recurring illnesses, crippling so valuable a life. What a satire it is to call our science "The Art of Healing"!

My provincial trip has been very interesting to me, as bringing me into contact with a great number of people in different classes of society, showing me everywhere a great want and an eager reception of what I have to give. From Leeds, Nottingham, and Edinburgh came earnest invitations to lecture. A message sent to my sister from Edinburgh stated a total revolution in womanly sentiment, and that her reception would now be as hearty as it was formerly hostile. A student from Cambridge told me the young men were warmly in our favour.

Mothers beg me for instruction in health. Young ladies listen eagerly to the idea of work. Three desired to become medical students. Wise old physicians ask me to "break up" certain fashionable London practices by substituting our own practice. Thus from many different points of view a deep interest awakens, but everywhere the London experience was repeated—viz. *conversion*; women thinking themselves hostile, but receiving the idea when they knew what it really meant. But the sympathy is necessarily intellectual only—practical reception and familiarity with the new position of women must necessarily be of slow growth. It must be, in fact, a life work. The children of the present generation will grow up accustomed to women doctors, respecting and trusting them, but the large majority of the adults will only hold a half-faith, and this will be a gradual growth. I am convinced that there would not be a rapidly brilliant success in England, such as some enthusiastic friends dream of.

There is a call for the work, an admirable field, but the work itself is a very slow one, the steady conquest of innumerable difficulties—a creation, in fact. The hospital scheme I think premature.

I had promised to bring it forward, and have done so, but I believe, to be successful, it must spring, as in America, out of private practice. I have no faith in its rapid success.

My own opinions and plans, then, may be briefly summed up.

There is a valuable and much-needed work to be done in England. Slow, uphill work, not remunerative (my tour was an expense to me); a repetition, to a great extent, of our last seven years' work. It would need us both to do it well; and so greatly does England want just our experience that, were it possible, I should counsel the transference of our work to this side of the water. But this we cannot do, and I shall therefore endeavour to prepare others for English work by receiving and educating students in America. In America, as here, it is a life work. I shall go back to create the institutions of which we have planted only the little germ. In ten years' time we may hope for permanent institutions there, worthy of their object, but we can during that time efficiently aid earnest young Englishwomen for their work here. Mrs. Bracebridge, who is much interested in this plan, is coming to London in Trinity Week for the special purpose of becoming acquainted with Mrs. Gurney and Mrs. Battin. They will form a committee for appointing and testing students. There will be a good deal of work connected with these arrangements, but directly it is completed I leave, as I am much wanted across the water.

I shall see you, my dear friend, before I leave (about June 25). I shall be sad to say good-bye, but I know that distance will not necessarily part us.

73 Gloucester Terrace, London: June 17, 1859.

DEAR E.,—I have only one piece of information to send, but that is of the highest importance—viz. that the Medical Council has registered me as physician! I have just learned the news from my lawyer, Mr. Shaen, who made the application, and at once forwarded the necessary fees, that I may be published in the first register. This will be of immeasurable value to the future of medical women in England. . . .

73 Gloucester Terrace: July 7.

I am busy making inquiries about the plates, &c., I want to take over to New York. I cannot go to the expense of a journey to Paris, but I have the catalogue of Auzoux, who stands unrivalled in the manufacture of *papier-mâché* models. I must make a selection and let the pieces be boxed up in Paris, and sent direct by sailing vessel. Vassourie is the modeller in wax; his models are the most exquisite things I have ever seen, but horribly dear. The microscope I shall buy in England I have settled to sail by the *Persia* on the 23rd, but the difficulty of deciding on our future course does not lessen. I am convinced that England is the place where we should work to best advantage. Lady Byron, Mrs. Bracebridge, the Peter Taylors, Miss Goldsmid—each the centre of a large and very different set of people—are each of them sure that we should have a large and valuable practice. Many doctors think the same. I cannot but think that the next ten years might be better spent in England than America. Our work is needed, and I know not who else can do it; indeed, we seem peculiarly suited to do this work in England. Well, we will soon discuss these matters together, and I am managing as well as I can in shaping things here, and gathering information under the uncertainty.

Returning to New York in August 1859, I found the permanent fund which had been commenced for the purchase of a hospital site prospering. The steady friends of the movement—Stacy B. Collins, Robert Haydock, Merritt Trimble, and Samuel Willets, formed the nucleus of an earnest band of supporters, both men and women. The spacious house, 126 Second Avenue, was purchased and adapted to the use of hospital and dispensary, with accommodation for several students.

Our able fellow-worker, Dr. Zackrzewska, having left us to superintend the new hospital in Boston, we carried on the rapidly growing work of the infirmary with the aid of intelligent graduates from Philadelphia, who came to us for practical instruction in medicine.

In addition to the usual departments of hospital and dispensary practice, which included the visiting of poor patients at their own homes, we established a sanitary visitor. This post was filled by one of our assistant physicians, whose special duty it was to give simple, practical instruction to poor mothers on the management of infants and the preservation of the health of their families. An intelligent young coloured physician, Dr. Cole, who was one of our resident assistants, carried on this work with tact and care. Experience of its results serve to show that the establishment of such a department would be a valuable addition to every hospital.

Correspondence with English friends continued, and we were deeply interested by the following letters from Miss Elizabeth Garrett, who was bravely commencing the necessary pioneer work in England:—

Aldeburgh, Suffolk: January 2, 1861.

I feel anxious to tell you how very much I enjoy the work and study, as this is to a great extent unexpected to me. As I had not any very strong interest in the subjects, and was led to choose the profession more from a strong conviction of its fitness for women than from any absorbing personal bias, I was prepared to find the first year's preparation work tedious and wearing. That this has not been the case is, I believe, mainly due to the fact of my having access to the hospital practice, which acts as a continual aid and stimulus to study. For three months I attended as a probationary nurse, learning what I could both from the doctors and nurses, and reading in the spare moments. It was, however, very difficult to make way in this desultory manner. The temptation to discursiveness and want of system met me continually, and at last I determined to begin the study of anatomy, chemistry, and materia medica, working steadily at these and enduring the ignorance of other branches which could not be studied rightly till a foundation of this kind had been laid. In pursuance of this plan, when the three months' nursing had expired I had an interview with the treasurer of the hospital, and asked permission to visit the wards and go round with the house doctors. This Mr. De Morgan agreed to, and also suggested that Mr. Plaskitt, the apothecary, should be asked to take me as a pupil in the dispensary, which I found him very willing to do. Mr. De Morgan, however, will hold out no hope of my being admitted as a regular student, and the general feeling seems to be that each doctor is willing to help me privately and singly, but they are afraid to countenance the movement by helping me in their collective capacity. This will, however, come in time, I trust, and in the meantime it is a great thing to meet with so much individual courtesy and help. When I left the special nursing work, Dr. Willis, the house physician, offered to superintend my reading in private lessons at my own house, which was precisely the kind of help I was most glad to accept. I continue to go to the hospital early, and go round the female medical wards alone, making notes of all difficulties and writing descriptions of heart and chest sounds and diagnosing as well as I can. This occupies the time till Dr. Willis comes, when I go round again and consult him upon all doubtful points, and learn a great deal by observing his method and principles. After this I go into the dispensary for two or three hours and learn the Pharmacopœia practically, and spend the afternoon in study in a room which the authorities have kindly lent me in the hospital. I am to continue on my present footing till April, but beyond that time I have no very clear plans. I wish to get all the education that is possible in London, even if it must be of a private or irregular kind. Perhaps it would be best to call upon Dr. Southwood Smith, Dr. Mayo, and Dr. Jenner, and hear if they can help me into any other medical school.

I should be very glad to know your opinion upon the plan of applying for admittance as a student at the Middlesex for the next winter session, and also what you would advise in the event of this being refused.

22 Manchester Square: May 8, 1862.

I have delayed writing, hoping that I might have at last some good news of success to give you; now, as this seems farther off than I had hoped it would be, I will delay no longer. I think Mrs. Russell Gurney wrote you that I was spending all my time just now in preparing for the matriculation examination of the University of London. I decided to make this the first step, in consequence of the experience last summer brought us. We then made three very careful and vigorous efforts to gain the admission of women into a medical school. Those we tried were the Middlesex, the Westminster, and the London Hospitals; and early in this year we attempted the Grosvenor Street School. I need not tell you we were in each case unsuccessful, though in one or two cases the adverse decision was gained by a very small majority of votes. In each case those gentlemen who opposed always urged as one ground for their doing so, that as the examining bodies were not prepared to admit women to their examinations, the school could not educate a woman to be an illegal practitioner, and that by doing so they would incur the certain risk of injuring the school in the eyes of the public without really aiding women. The medical papers also took up the same line. The "Lancet" was particularly anxious to point out that we were beginning at the wrong end, and that the first thing we should do was to settle the question of examination. I also had private information from several of the lecturers at the Middlesex that if I could matriculate at the London University and enter as a medical student for its examinations, my friends at their school would do all they could to get the adverse decision there altered. I therefore applied to the Apothecaries' Hall and to the College of Surgeons, asking the latter body if they would allow me to compete for the special diploma for midwifery which they now give. This was refused, with an intimation that the College would not in any way countenance the introduction of ladies into the medical profession. The application to the Hall was more fortunate; the question turned on a legal technicality, and was referred to counsel and finally decided in my favour. I must, of course, conform to all the ordinary regulations, but when I have done so I can obtain the licence to practise granted by that body. One of the regulations I have met without difficulty—viz. being apprenticed to a medical man for five years before the final examination. I had indentures made out as soon as I knew the decision. The second one (spending three years in a medical school in the United Kingdom) is more difficult: it is something to be able to say when applying for admission into a school that the Hall would examine me and give me its licence. Still, as the licence is not all that I want, I thought it better to make an effort at some university for the M.D. For many reasons it seems desirable to make the attempt at the London University. The medical examinations there are exceedingly good; the constitution of the body is of the most liberal description, and no residence is required nor any teaching given, so that the students would not be brought into any kind of contact till they met in the examination-room. Students of all kinds (whatever degree they may ultimately desire to take) are required to pass the matriculation examination in arts, and this includes the classics, natural philosophy, and mathematics, besides a modern language and the ordinary school subjects, history and geography, and is altogether an examination which would require a more liberal and careful education (in the case of girls) than is now generally given, even if the candidates never went in for the M.A. or B.A. degree. It was clear that the only chance of obtaining admission to the examinations generally lay in keeping the question on the widest, most general ground, advocating the claims of governesses and other women who required a good general examination, without introducing the question of medical degrees or the admission of women to any new professions. The university is about to have a new charter, and we therefore thought that this was the time to raise the question by praying the Senate to obtain the insertion of a clause expressly extending to women the benefits of their examinations. Before doing this we had submitted the present charter to the Attorney-General, and had had his opinion upon the power of the Senate to admit women upon its authority, as it is now drawn up. He thought they had no power to do so, and therefore there was no alternative but to ask for a new clause. In order to get some expression of the general feeling on the question, circulars similar to the one I send you were extensively distributed. More than 1,500 were sent out, and as a result we obtained a very respectable number of names as allies. Some of their letters were so cordial that we had extracts printed and sent to the members of the Senate with the list of names. The Vice-Chancellor and Mr. Grote were throughout most kindly ready to help us, and to give the proposal the full weight of their influence. The discussion at the Senate came on yesterday, and was a most lengthened and animated one; of twenty-one members present, ten were for, ten against, and one neutral. The Chancellor (Lord Granville) then had the casting-vote, and gave it against us.

I am exceedingly sorry, as this would have been fraught with such great benefit to many different classes of women, and would, I think, have been just the encouragement needed by girls when they leave school to keep them interested in their studies and out of the merely fashionable or domestic life they are so liable to fall into. It would also have been a great encouragement to parents, and would have made them more willing to let their daughters have time and opportunity for culture after they leave the schoolroom. These advantages would have been widely felt, and for professional women, whether governesses or physicians, the opportunity of being able to take a degree would have been invaluable. However, it is not to be had now; perhaps, when they are having another charter eight or ten years hence, we may try again and succeed. I do not imagine there is much chance of being able to do more at any other university in the United Kingdom than we can do here, so that I fear the possibility of ever obtaining an English degree as M.D. is a very remote one.

My notion now is to try to get into a school and obtain the Apothecaries' Hall licence. If this should prove possible, it would occupy between three and four years from next October. I should then wish to come to America and obtain the M.D. there, and then spend a year in Paris. I should be glad to know if you think I ought to make a point of getting the best M.D. diploma I can, either in America or on the Continent, if it should prove impossible to obtain one here, and if I *can* get the Apothecaries' licence. My own feeling is in favour of having the M.D.; though it should be a foreign one, I believe it would command more respect than the licence from the Hall would alone. I am fortunately able to choose to do whatever is most advisable, as I need not be in a hurry to enter upon the profession from pecuniary or any other motives, and I think I cannot aid the cause more soundly than by trying to do everything in the most thorough and exact way. It would be well, I think, to spend a good deal of time and strength on getting the very best diploma or certificate open to women. Should it prove to be quite impossible to get into a school, the licence from the Hall would not be within my reach. I must, in this case, rely entirely on foreign diplomas and on American schools. I shall not be too ready to admit this necessity, as I fear the advantage to the cause would be greatly diminished by the fact of my being educated in America.

I should be very glad to spend a year with you in the infirmary after having studied in a school here, but I should be very sorry to give up my English friends and interests for the whole period of study, if it can by any means be avoided. Still, if it cannot, I am ready to go on with the work. The time spent in study has been most pleasant, and I am more than ever convinced both that this special work is one which a woman may have a divine right to engage in, and that every single woman's life is both happier and more useful if she has an absorbing interest and pursuit. I shall be very glad to have your advice, when you can kindly find time to write to me. Believe me, yours sincerely,

E. GARRETT.

In the full tide of our medical activity in New York, with a growing private practice and increasing hospital claims, the great catastrophe of civil war overwhelmed the country and dominated every other interest.

The first shot at Fort Sumpter aroused the whole North, and the assassination of Lincoln enlisted the indignant energy of every Northern woman in the tremendous struggle. As the deadly contest proceeded, and every town and village sent forth its volunteers to the fearful slaughter of civil war, the concentration of thought and action on the war dwarfed every other effort.

The war was essentially a rebellion by a portion of the States for the maintenance of slavery. To us, nourished from childhood on the idea of human freedom and justice, the contest became of absorbing interest. Though our American friends often reproached us as Englishwomen for the action of the English Government, we threw ourselves energetically into the cause of freedom.

On the outbreak of the war, an informal meeting of the lady managers was called at the infirmary to see what could be done towards supplying the want of trained nurses so widely felt after the first battles. A notice of this meeting to be held at the infirmary having accidentally found its way into the "New York Times," the parlours of the infirmary were crowded with ladies, to the surprise of the little group of managers.

The Rev. Dr. Bellows and Dr. Elisha Harris being present, a formal meeting was organised. Whilst the great and urgent need of a supply of nurses was fully recognised, it was also felt that the movement would be too vast to be carried on by so small an institution. A letter was therefore drafted on this occasion, calling for a public meeting at the Cooper Institute, and a committee of the ladies present was appointed to obtain signatures to this call.

The meeting at the Cooper Institute was crowded to overflowing. The National Sanitary Aid Association was then formed, in order to organise the energetic efforts to help that were being made all over the country.

The Ladies' Sanitary Aid Association, of which we were active members, was also formed. This branch worked daily at the Cooper Institute during the whole of the war. It received and forwarded contributions of comforts for the soldiers, zealously sent from the country; but its special work was the forwarding of nurses to the seat of war. All that could be done in the extreme urgency of the need was to sift out the most promising women from the multitudes that applied to be sent on as nurses, put them for a month in training at the great Bellevue Hospital of New York, which consented to receive relays of volunteers, provide them with a small outfit, and send them on for distribution to Miss Dix, who was appointed superintendent of nurses at Washington.

The career of one of these nurses, a German, deserves recording. We hesitated about receiving her, on account of her excitable disposition, but she insisted on going. This feeble-looking woman soon drifted away from the Washington Depôt to the active service of the front. After the battle of Gettysburg she spent two days and nights on the field of slaughter, wading with men's boots in the blood and mud, pulling out the still living bodies from the heaps of slain, binding up hideous wounds, giving a draught of water to one, placing a rough pillow under the head of another, in an enthusiasm of beneficence which triumphed equally over thought of self and horror of the hideous slaughter.

A welcome relief to the great tension of life during those years was the visit of Mr. Herman Bicknell, F.R.C.S., who was travelling in America after the death of his wife. I remembered him as a fellow-student of the St. Bartholomew's days, who sat by me in the lecture-room; and he recalled many interesting reminiscences of that eventful time. He was a man of great though eccentric talent, and a clever Persian scholar, having resided long in the East. His cordial friendship during many later years was much prized, and continued until his premature death.

It was not until this great national rebellion was ended that the next step in the growth of the infirmary could be taken.

The infirmary service of young assistant physicians, which had been hitherto supplied by students whose theoretical training had been obtained elsewhere, no longer met the New York needs.

In 1865 the trustees of the infirmary, finding that the institution was established in public favour, applied to the Legislature for a charter conferring college powers upon it.

They took this step by the strong advice of some of the leading physicians of New York interested in the infirmary, who urged that the medical education of women should not be allowed to pass into the hands of the irresponsible persons who were at that time seeking to establish a women's college in New York. We took this step, however, with hesitation, for our own feeling was adverse to the formation of an entirely separate school for women. The first women physicians connected with the infirmary, having all been educated in the ordinary medical schools, felt very strongly the advantage of admission to the large organised system of public instruction already existing for men; and also the benefits arising from association with men as instructors and companions in the early years of medical study. They renewed their efforts, therefore, to induce some good recognised New York school to admit, under suitable arrangements, a class of students guaranteed by the infirmary, rather than add another to the list of female colleges already existing. Finding, however, after consultation with the different New York schools, that such arrangements could not at present be made, the trustees followed the advice of their consulting staff, obtained a college charter, and opened a subscription for a college fund.

The use of a spacious lecture-room in the New York University, on Washington Square, was temporarily obtained, until the house adjoining the infirmary could be leased and fitted for college purposes.[1]

1. The fine property on Stuyvesant Square, at the corner of East Fifteenth Street, has since been purchased, and is now the site of the New York Infirmary and College.

A full course of college instruction was gradually organised, with the important improvement of establishing the subject of hygiene as one of the principal professorial chairs, thus making it an equal as well as obligatory study. Another important improvement adopted was the establishment of an Examination Board, independent of the teaching staff, a plan not then customary in the United States. This Board was composed of some of the best known members of the profession, and at the same time we changed the ordinary term of medical study from three years to four.

During the early years of the college I occupied the Chair of Hygiene, and had the pleasure of welcoming Miss Jex Blake, then visiting America, as a member of the first class. The Professor of Hygiene also superintended the important work of the sanitary visitor at the homes of the poor. It has always seemed to me, during many years of active private practice, that the first and constant aim of the family physician should be to diffuse the sanitary knowledge which would enable parents to bring up healthy children.

The most painful experience which I met with in practice was the death of one of my little patients from the effects of vaccination. This baby, though carefully tended and the lymph used guaranteed pure, died from the phagedenic ulceration set up by vaccination in a rather scrofulous constitution. To a hygienic physician thoroughly believing in the beneficence of Nature's laws, to have caused the death of a child by such means was a tremendous blow!

This serious experience awakened a growing distrust as to the wisdom of all medical methods which introduce any degree of morbid matter into the blood of the human system; a distrust which no amount of temporary professional opinion or doubtful statistics has been able to remove. Although I have always continued to vaccinate when desired, I am strongly opposed to every form of inoculation of attenuated virus, as an unfortunate though well-meaning fallacy of medical prejudice.

Chapter Seven

Return to England

1869

IN 1869 the early pioneer work in America was ended. During the twenty years which followed the graduation of the first woman physician, the public recognition of the justice and advantage of such a measure had steadily grown. Throughout the Northern States the free and equal entrance of women into the profession of medicine was secured. In Boston, New York, and Philadelphia special medical schools for women were sanctioned by the Legislatures, and in some long-established colleges women were received as students in the ordinary classes.

Our New York centre was well organised under able guidance, and I determined to return to England for a temporary though prolonged residence, both to renew physical strength, which had been severely tried, and to enlarge my experience of life, as well as to assist in the pioneer work so bravely commencing in London, and which extended later to Edinburgh.

I soon found that social questions of vital importance to

human progress were taking root in the prepared soil of the older civilisation—questions which were of absorbing interest. During the following twenty years the responsibility of the Christian physician assumed to me an ever-deepening significance.

After a refreshing tour in the lovely Lake District, arranged by my old friend Herman Bicknell, we attended the Social Science Congress held in Bristol in September of 1869. This was indeed a noteworthy experience. I was the guest with Miss Mary Carpenter of her relations Mr. and Mrs. Thomas. One morning Miss Carpenter came into my room with her hands full of papers, saying, "These papers refer to a subject that you must take up. It is to be discussed at a sectional meeting to-day, from which all women are excluded; but you, as a doctor, have a right to be present, and will be admitted, and you *must* attend."

This formed my introduction to that tremendous campaign against the unequal standard of sexual morality known as the repeal of the "Contagious Diseases Acts," in which for the following seventeen years I was to take an active part, and which, from its extended bearings, moulded the whole of my future life.

The study of the papers thus brought to my notice by Miss Carpenter was a revelation to me. Perhaps happily for me, during my past life and medical experiences I had never fully realised the wide bearing of this subject and the inevitable social degradation produced by a double standard of morality. My eyes were now suddenly opened, never to be closed again, to that direful purchase of women which is really the greatest obstacle to the progress of the race.

Ignorant as I then was of the various aspects of the Contagious Diseases Acts, I instantly perceived their injustice, and at once accepted the difficult mission Miss Carpenter laid upon me.

It was hoped by some members of the congress that a resolution would be passed supporting the one-sided Contagious Diseases Acts legislation, against which a strong opposition was beginning to arise, and I resolved that the voice of one member of the congress, at any rate, should support the foundation of morality—viz. equal justice. I therefore attended the section, held at the Blind Asylum, sitting far back in that assemblage of men.

I soon found, however, to my immense relief and gratitude, that the cause of justice was in able and vigorous male hands, led by Professor Francis Newman; so I gladly withdrew from a painful position in that sectional meeting, my advocacy not being needed.

I was privileged at this time to make the acquaintance of the Rev. Charles Kingsley and his generous-hearted wife. On our first meeting, at an evening party, Mr. Kingsley overwhelmed me by his enthusiastic greeting. "You are one of my heroes," he said—a speech which I really could not then understand; it seemed to stun me, in my quiet life. Later, as I learned to know his enthusiastic character and profound social insight, I knew his meaning. A sincere personal friendship was then begun. He supported me by constant and wise counsel until the time of his lamented death, which was indeed a severe personal loss. I was warmly welcomed to the Rectory of Eversley, and later to the Deanery of Chester. On the pleasant and historic pine hills of Bramshill, by the Eversley Parsonage, and on the ancient walls of Chester, with their noble outlook to the Welsh mountains, when visiting the Deanery, I enjoyed memorable walks with this generous-hearted man, when he threw open his delightful stores of natural history and strengthened me by his social wisdom.

An amusing personal experience at the Bristol Congress was

a "breakfast of all the religions," organised by my eccentric friend Herman Bicknell, and at which he insisted that I should help him preside. He said to me: "Holyoake is an Atheist, Cowell Stepney a Materialist, Baunerjé and Chatterjé are of the Hindoo Brahma Somaj, you are a Christian, and I am a Catholic. It will be a most remarkable gathering, and the discussion of such varied opinions extremely interesting." I accepted the queer invitation. The breakfast was held in a large parlour of the hotel. We assembled at table, and one of the first things the very deaf gentleman on my right hand said to me was: "What an extraordinary, odd notion that of a soul is! I wonder how it could have arisen." But the most interesting remark by far was made by Holyoake, who, returning from a secularist meeting of Bristol working men, was at once accosted by our host: "Now, Holyoake, pray let us have your famous demonstration of the non-existence of a God." Mr. Holyoake accepted the demand, and thought for some time in a profound silence; then, with a puzzled face, he suddenly burst out: "Upon my word, Bicknell, I have really quite forgotten it!"

Mr. Kingsley once said to me, pointing to Holyoake: "That man, many years ago, I put into prison for blasphemy; now I am begging him to come down and visit me at Eversley!" Our breakfast of all the religions as an active contest was a failure. The hostile forces met together, but, instead of fighting, they fraternised!

It was during this visit to Bristol in 1869 that the curious experience, already referred to on page [54], occurred, when I visited the house where my early childhood was spent.

On settling in London as a physician, I resided for some time with my valued friend Barbara Leigh Smith, then Madame Bodichon, at whose house in Blandford Square I met her wide and varied circle of literary and artistic friends and many leaders of social reform. Herbert Spencer, Dante Rossetti, Mrs. Lewes, the Peter Taylors, Mrs. Crawshay, Miss Goldsmid, Miss Cobbe, and Keshub Chunder Sen represent a few of the persons I was privileged to meet.

At this time I had engaged medical consultation-rooms in an apparently respectable house in York Place, on the front door of which the house agent allowed me to place my name. I soon found, however, that my doctor's sign was intended to conceal the dubious character of the occupier of the house, and I had unconsciously walked into a trap! But friends came to the rescue and compelled the cancelling of the lease with which I was entangled. I then established myself at No. 6 Burwood Place, where the commencement of a promising medical practice was soon formed.

I eagerly entered upon the varied and intensely interesting social life now opened to me.

My long-cherished conviction of the supreme importance of the medical profession as the great conservator of health constantly deepened.

In 1870, being invited to address the Working Women's College, I took as the subject of my discourse "How to Keep a Household in Health." This lecture laid down rules of health for the guidance of poor women in the management of their households, and was welcomed by the audience. One person present, however, sent a slanderous account of this lecture to the "Pall Mall Gazette," and I was overwhelmed by the receipt of anonymous letters, and letters from persons in all classes of society, requesting medical advice on the most important and delicate subjects—subjects which are only suitable for the confidential counsel of the physician's consulting-room, where alone advice adapted to each individual case can be judiciously given. I mentioned this experience of the newspaper attack and the subsequent correspondence to my friend Mr. Kingsley. He exclaimed: "Oh, you did not answer those letters, I trust?" I assured him that I had always refused to give the advice asked for by letter, and had invariably returned fees when enclosed. "Thank God for that!" he exclaimed with an energy that amazed me; and he then related to me a very painful experience of his own, saying: "Let me warn you, never answer a newspaper attack. There are some newspapers that delight in getting hold of a scandal or whatever may make their paper sell, and are utterly unscrupulous as to the means by which such a purpose is accomplished. You have no chance against such corrupt speculation; your only weapon is silence and your own established character."

On February 19, 1871, under the auspices of the Sunday Lecture Society, I gave an address, "On the Religion of Health," to a large appreciative audience in St. George's Hall. The same year a small meeting was held in the drawing-room of 6 Burwood Place, to consider the important subject of a steady and wide diffusion of sanitary knowledge among all the people. There "The National Health Society" was formed, for which Mr. Prout Newcombe (who was present) shaped the stamp of the society, with its motto, "Prevention is better than cure." This society, which established its first office in Berners Street under the intelligent secretaryship of Miss Toulmin Smith, continues its enlarging sphere of usefulness under the able management of Miss Fay Lankester.

At this time the medical dispensary established by Miss Garrett for women and children in Seymour Place was growing and enlisting a large number of influential friends.

From this small beginning has grown the New Hospital and London School of Medicine for Women, connected with the Royal Free Hospital. This is not the place to speak of the intelligent and persevering efforts to which those institutions owe their origin. The work of Dr. Garrett Anderson and Dr. Sophia Jex Blake will always be remembered. It was my privilege and pleasure in some small degree to encourage these brave workers in their pioneer enterprise in England.

Whilst attending to an increasing medical practice, a visit from Mr. William Pare, who had written an interesting account of the Ralahine land experiment in Ireland, which proved so successful under the management of Mr. E. T. Craig, drew my attention to the important co-operative movement steadily growing in England.[1] The abortive attempts at co-operative society which I had watched in the United States, at Brook Farm, Red Bank, Eagleswood, and other places, in no way shook the faith that through failure and renewed effort the true principles of a wise organisation of human relations would gradually be evolved. The English co-operative movement was characteristic of the common-sense, unambitious way in which reforms grow in England. The religious element introduced by such a noble band of Christian Socialists as Maurice, Kingsley, Hughes, and Ludlow gave a hopefulness to this movement which no attempts based on a limited view of material well-being can afford.

Medical experience was daily showing the influence of the mind over the body, and I eagerly longed to see an embodiment of Christian principles in society, which embodiment was, as yet, far from attainment.

1. This remarkable experiment of 1831, with its tragic termination, is related by Mr. Pare (Longmans, Green, & Co.) and by Mr. Craig (Trübner). It is well worth the careful study of all co-operative reformers.

In pursuance of this investigation, at the end of August 1872 I determined to visit the Familistère of Guise, formed by Godin Lemaire. His book, "Solutions Sociales," describing the growth of the institution, was exceedingly interesting, and contained valuable suggestions for future workers, and I wished to see its practical working for myself. At the end of a fatiguing journey to Guise, on the Belgian frontier of France, for at that time many miles had to be traversed by diligence, I was cordially welcomed by M. Lemaire, and spent several very interesting days in the great Familistère, observing the life there.

The Familistère, which accommodated several hundred people, was erected on a tract of land almost encircled by the river, which tract was laid out in gardens and pleasure grounds. Across the river stood the large factories and workshops for the manufacture of stoves, &c., which furnished the remunerative occupation of the little community.

I attended the prize-giving at the schools, saw the theatre, workmen's club and choral society, witnessed a ball, and visited the manufactory. The organisation was a great object-lesson both in its success and its defects; full of interest to those who seriously study this important subject of improved social relations. The life at the Familistère, however, was intense, and rather overpowering to me.

Shortly after my return I was attacked by illness, which proved so serious in its effects that in 1873 the Burwood Place establishment was broken up, and my plan of life necessarily changed. During the next three years I vainly endeavoured to resume my London work, but was frequently obliged to seek health in change of residence and foreign travel. This travel included a memorable winter in Rome, which need not be further referred to, although the approach to the Eternal City—

when, across the Campagna, the dome of St. Peter's was first visible—was a thrilling personal joy, never to be forgotten. But my purely personal experiences will not be dwelt on.

When the London School of Medicine for Women was established I hastened my return, and accepted the Chair of Gynæcology in the college.

In my lodgings in Dorset Square I again suffered from atrocious biliary colic, which the able physicians whom I consulted were unable to relieve, finished my course of lectures with extreme difficulty, and came to the conclusion, with bitter disappointment, that any future residence in London under my circumstances must be given up.

The winters of 1876–78 were spent chiefly at Bordighera and in Nice. An episode there is worth recording.

My enlarging experience in various countries in respect to the relations between men and women—the customs, the diseases, the social disaster springing from errors as to human physiology and neglect in education with regard to the most important functions—showed me the imperative work which devolved upon the physician in this matter. I realised that the mind cannot be separated from the body in any profound view of the scope of medical responsibility. Under the olive trees of Bordighera, and sitting by its lovely blue sea, I meditated on the duty of the physician, and finally wrote the small work, "Counsel to Parents on the Moral Education of their Children."

So little at that time was the importance of sexual education understood, and the necessity of its consideration accepted, that when I read my manuscript to a warm and enlightened English friend staying at Mentone, she assured me that if I published that manuscript my "name would be a forbidden word in England."

I sent the manuscript, however, to about twelve of the leading London publishers, who all declined the publication. I therefore printed a small edition myself, which a bookseller consented to keep on sale. A copy of this little book fell under the notice of Miss Ellice Hopkins, who, considering that it would be useful in the special work in which she was engaged, induced Mr. Hudson, the then acting member of the firm of Hatchard & Co., to reconsider the matter and publish the book for her use. The arrangement was made and the book printed; but soon after I received a letter saying that though the firm had never yet broken faith with an author, yet they feared they must do so now; for the senior member of the firm, Bishop Hatchard's widow, had seen the proof of the book, thrown it into the fire, and desired that its publication should be stopped!

Finally, a little consultation of elderly clergymen was called to consider the subject, and it was at last resolved that if the name of the work could be changed, and the distinct announcement made in the title that it was a medical as well as a moral work, the publication might be continued. Of course the change was made, and "Counsel to Parents" became "The Moral Education of the Young, considered under *Medical* and Social Aspects."

I mention this curious experience as an encouragement to those who are engaged in all branches of moral work. Public sentiment has advanced since 1876. Looking now at the very reticent way in which the subject is treated in this little book, it is difficult to believe that such an episode could have occurred.

It has become clear to me that our medical profession has not yet fully realised the special and weighty responsibility which rests upon it to watch over the cradle of the race; to see that human beings are well born, well nourished, and well educated. The onward impulse to this great work would seem to be especially incumbent upon women physicians, who for the first time are beginning to realise the all-important character of parentage in its influence upon the adult as well as on the child—i.e. on the race.

To every woman, as well as to every man, the responsible function of parentage is delegated. Our nature is dwarfed or degraded if the growth which should be attained by the exercise of parentage, directly or potentially, be either avoided or perverted.

The physician knows that the natural family group is the first essential element of a progressive society. The degeneration of that element by the degradation of either of its two essential factors, the man or the woman, begins the ruin of a State.

It is a source of deep gratitude in a long medical life to have been enabled by physiological knowledge, as well as experience, to perceive the true point of view from which the special nature of man and woman must be regarded. It is well worth the efforts of a lifetime to have attained knowledge which justifies an attack on the root of all evil—viz. the deadly atheism which asserts that because forms of evil have always existed in society, therefore they must always exist; and that the attainment of a high ideal is a hopeless chimera.

The study of human nature by women as well as men commences that new and hopeful era of the intelligent co-operation of the sexes through which alone real progress can be attained and secured. We may look forward with hope to the future influence of Christian women physicians, when with sympathy and reverence guiding intellectual activity they learn to apply the vital principles of their Great Master to every method and practice of the healing art.

Appendix

I

THE following letter, lately published in the New York "Church Union" by a well-known physician of New York, is interesting as the testimony of a gentleman who was a fellow-student in the Geneva Medical College.

THE MEDICAL CO-EDUCATION OF THE SEXES. BY STEPHEN SMITH, M.D.

Medical circles were recently entertained by a symposium of prominent physicians discussing the propriety of the medical co-education of the sexes. All of the writers were opposed to the suggestion; some, notably Dr. Weir Mitchell, of Philadelphia, expressed the utmost disgust at the proposition. It happened to me to have witnessed the first instance of the co-education of medical students of both sexes in this country, and the results quite upset the theories of these gentlemen.

The first course of medical lectures which I attended was in a medical college in the interior of this State in 1847–48. The class, numbering about 150 students, was composed largely of young men from the neighbouring towns. They were rude, boisterous, and riotous beyond comparison. On several occasions the residents of the neighbourhood sent written protests to the faculty, threatening to have the college indicted as a nuisance if the disturbance did not cease. During lectures it was often almost impossible to hear the professors, owing to the confusion.

Some weeks after the course began the dean appeared before the class with a letter in his hand, which he craved the indulgence of the students to be allowed to read. Anticipation was extreme when he announced that it contained the most extraordinary request which had ever been made to the faculty. The letter was written by a physician of Philadelphia, who requested the faculty to admit as a student a lady who was studying medicine in his office. He stated that she had been refused admission by several medical colleges, but, as this institution was in the country, he thought it more likely to be free from prejudice against a woman medical student. The dean stated that the faculty had taken action on the communication, and directed him to report their conclusion to the class. The faculty decided to leave the matter in the hands of the class, with this understanding—that if any single student objected to her admission, a negative reply would be returned. It subsequently appeared that the faculty did not intend to admit her, but wished to escape direct refusal by referring the question to the class, with a proviso which, it was believed, would necessarily exclude her.

But the whole affair assumed the most ludicrous aspect to the class, and the announcement was received with the most uproarious demonstrations of favour. A meeting was called for the evening, which was attended by every member. The resolution approving the admission of the lady was sustained by a number of the most extravagant speeches, which were enthusiastically cheered. The vote was finally taken, with what seemed to be one unanimous yell, "Yea!" When the negative vote was called, a single voice was heard uttering a timid "No." The scene that followed passes description. A general rush was made for the corner of the room which emitted the voice, and the recalcitrant member was only too glad to acknowledge his error and record his vote in the affirmative. The faculty received the decision of the class with evident disfavour, and returned an answer admitting the lady student. Two weeks or more elapsed, and as the lady student did not appear, the incident of her application was quite forgotten, and the class continued in its riotous career. One morning, all unexpectedly, a lady entered the lecture-room with the professor; she was quite small of stature, plainly dressed, appeared diffident and retiring, but had a firm and determined expression of face. Her entrance into that Bedlam of confusion acted like magic upon every student. Each hurriedly sought his seat, and the most absolute silence prevailed. For the first time a lecture was given without the slightest interruption, and every word could be heard as distinctly as it would if there had been but a single person in the room. The sudden transformation of this class from a band of lawless desperadoes to gentlemen, by the mere presence of a lady, proved to be permanent in its effects. A more orderly class of medical students was never seen than this, and it continued to be to the close of the term.

The real test of the influence of a woman upon the conduct and character of a man in co-education was developed when the Professor of Anatomy came to that part of his course which required demonstrations that he believed should be witnessed only by men. The professor was a rollicking, jovial man, who constantly interspersed his lectures with witty remarks and funny anecdotes. Nor did he study to have his language chaste, or the moral of his stories pure and elevating. In fact, vulgarity and profanity formed a large part of his ordinary lectures; and especially was this true of the lectures on the branch of anatomy above mentioned. On this account, chiefly, he was exceedingly popular with his class; and during his lectures stamping, clapping, and cheering were the principal employments of the students.

One morning our lady student was missed at the lecture on anatomy, and the professor entered the room evidently labouring under great excitement. He stated that he had a communication to make to the class which demanded the most serious consideration. He then explained that he had thought it highly improper that the lady student should attend certain lectures specially adapted for men, and as he was approaching that subject he had frankly advised her to absent herself, in a letter which he read. He dwelt upon the indelicacy of the subject, the embarrassment under which he should labour if a lady were present, and the injustice which would be done to the class by the imperfect manner in which he should be obliged to demonstrate the subject. He closed by offering her abundant private opportunities for study and dissection. He then read her reply. It was gracefully written, and showed a full appreciation of his embarrassing position, when viewed from the low standpoint of impure and unchaste sentiments. But she could not conceive of a medical man whose mind was not so elevated and purified by the study of the science of anatomy that such sentiments would for a moment influence him. Coming to the practical question of her attendance upon these lectures, she stated that if the professor would really be embarrassed by the presence of a lady on the first tier of seats, she would take her seat on the upper tier; and she trusted that his interest in his subject would lead him to entirely forget the presence of student No. 130—her registered number. At the close of the letter the professor acknowledged the justice of the rebuke which he had received, and declared that a lady who was animated by such elevated views of her profession was entitled to every possible encouragement which the class or faculty could give. He then opened the door and she entered, only to receive an ovation of the most overwhelming character. The lectures on anatomy proceeded in regular order to their conclusion; and it was the universal testimony of the oldest students that they had never listened to such a complete and thorough course.

At the close of the term our lady student came up for examination for graduation, and took rank with the best students of the class. As this was the first instance of the granting of a medical diploma to a woman in this country, so far as the faculty had information, there was at first some hesitation about conferring the degree. But it was finally determined to take the novel step, and in the honour list of the roll of graduates for that year appears the name, Dr. Elizabeth Blackwell.

Church Union.

New York, 1892.

II

AN M.D. IN A GOWN

[The "Medical Times" of the 21st ult. contains a full, true, and particular account of the admission of a young lady, Miss Elizabeth Blackwell, by the General Medical College, in the State of New York, to a physician's degree. Miss Blackwell had duly attended lectures at the college, and received a formal diploma, under the title of "Domina," which was the only feminine that the Senate could find for Doctor. "Punch" really thinks this is a case for a copy of verses, which he accordingly subjoins, in honour of the fair M.D.]

Not always is the warrior male,
 Nor masculine the sailor;
We all know Zaragossa's tale,

We've all heard "Billy Taylor";
But far a nobler heroine, she
Who won the palm of knowledge,
And took a Medical Degree,
By study at her College.

They talk about the gentler sex
Mankind in sickness tending,
And o'er the patient's couch their necks
Solicitously bending;
But what avails solicitude
In fever or in phthisic,
If lovely woman's not imbued
With one idea of physic?

Young ladies all, of every clime,
Especially of Britain,
Who wholly occupy your time
In novels or in knitting,
Whose highest skill is but to play,
Sing, dance, or French to clack well,
Reflect on the example, pray,
Of excellent Miss Blackwell!

Think, if you had a brother ill,
A husband, or a lover,
And could prescribe the draught or pill
Whereby he might recover;
How much more useful this would be,
Oh, sister, wife, or daughter!
Than merely handing him beef-tea,
Gruel, or toast-and-water.

Ye bachelors about to wed
    In youth's unthinking hey-day,
Who look upon a furnish'd head
    As horrid for a lady,
Who'd call a female doctor "blue";
    You'd spare your sneers, I rather
Think, my young fellows, if you knew
    What physic costs a father!

How much more blest were married life
    To men of small condition,
If every one could have his wife
    For family physician;
His nursery kept from ailments free,
    By proper regulation,
And for advice his only fee
    A thankful salutation.

For Doctrix Blackwell—that's the way
    To dub in rightful gender—
In her profession, ever may
    Prosperity attend her!
"Punch" a gold-handled parasol
    Suggests for presentation
To one so well deserving all
    Esteem and admiration.

1849.

III

FIRST ANNUAL REPORT OF THE NEW YORK DISPENSARY FOR POOR WOMEN AND CHILDREN, 1855

The design of this institution is to give to poor women an opportunity of consulting physicians of their own sex. The existing charities of our city regard the employment of women as physicians as an experiment, the success of which has not yet been sufficiently proved to admit of cordial co-operation. It was therefore necessary to form a separate institution which should furnish to poor women the medical aid which they could not obtain elsewhere.

The following gentlemen cordially consented to act as trustees of the proposed institution: Messrs. Butler, White, Haydock, Sedgwick, Collins, Field, Draper, Greeley, West, Harris, Foster, Raymond, Flanders, Dana, Manning, Spring, Bowne. Consulting physicians, Drs. Kissam, Parker, Cammann, Taylor. Attending physician, Dr. Elizabeth Blackwell.

Messrs. Sedgwick and Butler kindly procured an Act of Incorporation. A meeting for organisation was held on January 30, 1854. A constitution and bylaws were adopted, and the following members were appointed an Executive Committee to transact the business for the year: Stacy B. Collins, Richard H. Bowne, Charles A. Dana, Elizabeth Blackwell, Charles Foster.

The Eleventh Ward was chosen as the location for the dispensary, it being destitute of medical charity, while possessing a densely crowded poor population. The necessary rooms were found in Seventh Street, near Tompkins Square, and were ready for the reception of patients in the month of March. The dispensary has been regularly opened through the year, on Monday, Wednesday, and Friday afternoons, at 3 o'clock. Over 200 poor women have received medical aid. All these women have gratefully acknowledged the help afforded them, and several of the most destitute have tendered their few pence as an offering to the institution.

With all these patients, the necessity of cleanliness, ventilation, and judicious diet has been strongly urged, and in many cases the advice has been followed, at any rate for a time. A word of counsel or information, too, has often been given to the destitute widow or friendless girl who was seeking work as well as health; the best methods of seeking employment have been pointed out, suitable charities occasionally recommended, and pecuniary aid sometimes rendered.

Since the double distress of commercial pressure and severe weather have weighed so heavily on the poor, many cases of extreme destitution have come to the dispensary. These have been chiefly emigrants, mostly Germans, without friends or money, and ignorant of the language. Several families have been visited where some member was sick, and found utterly destitute, suffering from hunger, and though honest and industrious, disappointed in every effort to obtain work. To such families a little help with money, generally in the form of a loan till work could be procured, has proved invaluable, and a small poor fund placed by some friends in the hands of the attending physician, for this special object, has saved several worthy families from despair and impending starvation.

The dispensary has been removed since January 1, 1855, to No. 150 Third Street, between Avenues A and B, opposite the large Catholic church; all persons who are interested in its objects are cordially invited to call there. It will be open as heretofore from 3 to 5 o'clock on Monday, Wednesday, and Friday afternoons. Poor women and children may be sent from any part of the city to receive the medical aid of the dispensary, it being free to all.

This institution was commenced by the subscriptions of a few friends; its expenses have been kept within its means, but the power of doing good has necessarily been limited by the smallness of its funds. It is found desirable to enlarge its operations, and place it on a permanent basis. For this purpose, the trustees wish to raise the sum of 5,000 dollars, and contributions are earnestly solicited. The following members are appointed to receive contributions:

Stacy B. Collins, 155 Bleecker Street,
Robert Haydock, 46 Broadway,
Elizabeth Blackwell, 79 East Fifteenth Street.

The amount raised will be invested as a permanent fund for the institution. It is the hope of the founders of this charity to make it eventually a hospital for women and a school for the education of nurses.

The books of the dispensary are always open to the inspection of members, on application to the attending physician.

New York: February 8, 1855.

Bibliography

ADDRESSES

The following addresses and publications indicate that search after righteousness which has occupied later life in England.

How to keep a Household in Health; given at the Working Women's College, 1870.

Medicine and Morality, 1881; in the "Modern Review."

Rescue Work in relation to Vice and Disease, 1881; before Mrs. Meredith's Society.

Christian Socialism, 1882.

Wrong and Right Methods of dealing with Social Evil, based on Parliamentary Evidence, 1883.

On the Decay of Municipal Representative Government: a Personal Experience in Hastings, 1885.

Purchase of Women a Great Economic Blunder, 1886.

Criticism of Gronlund's Co-operative Commonwealth; given before the Fellowship of the New Life, 1888.

A Medical Treatise on the Corruption of Neo-Malthusianism, 1888.

Christian Duty in regard to Vice; a letter to the International Congress, 1889.

Christianity a Battle, not a Dream; given before the Christo-Theosophical Society.

Erroneous Method in Medical Education; Counsel to the Medical College of the New York Infirmary, 1892.

PUBLICATIONS

The Moral Education of the Young. (Longmans, Green & Co.)

The Human Element in Sex; a Medical Work. (J. & A. Churchill.)

Christianity in Medicine; published in "Things to Come." (Elliot Stock.)

The Influence of Women in Medicine; an Address to the Graduates of the London School of Medicine for Women. (Bell & Sons.)

Why Hygienic Congresses fail. (Bell & Sons.)

The Religion of Health; republished by the M. R. Union, 2 Leinster Place, W.

www.ingramcontent.com/pod-product-compliance
Ingram Content Group UK Ltd.
Pitfield, Milton Keynes, MK11 3LW, UK
UKHW012034150926
475560UK00001B/2

9 781538 179628